WORKBOOK

T0290273

2025

BUCK'S STEP-BY-STEP Medical Coding

Jackie L. Koesterman, CPC
Lead Technical Collaborator
Coding and Reimbursement Specialist
JDK Medical Coding EDU
Grand Forks, North Dakota

ELSEVIER

Elsevier
3251 Riverport Lane
St. Louis, Missouri 63043

BUCK'S WORKBOOK FOR STEP-BY-STEP MEDICAL CODING, 2025 EDITION
ISBN: 978-0-443-24879-5

NOTE: The 2025 *ICD-10-CM* and 2025 *ICD-10-PCS* were used in updating this text.

NOTE: *Current Procedural Terminology, 2025,* was used in updating this text.

Previous editions copyrighted 2024, 2023, 2022, 2021, 2020, 2019, 2018, 2017, 2016, 2015, 2014, 2013, 2012, 2011, 2010, 2009, 2008, 2007, 2006, 2005, 2004, and 2002.

Senior Content Strategist: Luke E. Held
Content Development Manager: Danielle Frazier
Senior Content Development Specialist: Joshua S. Rapplean
Publishing Services Manager: Deepthi Unni
Project Manager: Nayagi Anandan
Senior Book Designer: Maggie Reid

Printed in the United States of America

Last digit is the print number: 9 8 7 6 5 4 3 2 1

Preface

LET THIS BE YOUR GOAL:

People who have accomplished worthwhile [goals] have had a very high sense of the way to do things. They have not been content with mediocrity. They have not confined themselves to the beaten tracks; they have never been satisfied to do things just as others do them, but always a little better. They always pushed things that came to their hands a little higher up, a little farther on. It is this little higher up, this little farther on, that counts in the quality of life's work. It is the constant effort to be first class in everything one attempts that conquers the heights of excellence.

Orison Swett Marden

This *Workbook* has been developed to assist you in the application of the theoretical and practical coding knowledge presented in the textbook *Step-by-Step Medical Coding*. The *Workbook* parallels the textbook with presentation of Chapters 1 through 27 and includes ample opportunity to practice the skill of medical coding. The *Workbook* contains three levels of questions—theory, abbreviated patient service and diagnosis descriptions, and original reports. The first level of question is the theory question; these questions are fill-in-the-blanks, multiple choice, true or false, and matching and often include medical terminology based on the specific area of coding presented in the coding manuals. The theory information serves as the foundational knowledge necessary to correctly code services and diagnoses. The second level of question is the abbreviated patient service and diagnosis descriptions; these questions begin the practical application of coding. The descriptions are condensed statements that provide broad-based coding experience. The final level is presented at the end of most *Workbook* chapters and contains reports that represent more complex services and diagnosis descriptions, such as operative, pathology, radiology, and emergency services.

The format for the answers has been developed to guide you in the development of your coding ability by using a format that includes four response variations:

- **One answer blank** for coding questions that require one code for the answer.
- **Multiple answer blanks** for coding questions that require more than one code for the answer.
- Key terms next to the blank(s) to guide you through the most difficult coding scenarios.
- **Answer blanks with preceding the blank to indicate that you must decide the number of codes necessary to correctly answer the question.**

Appendix B of the *Workbook* contains the answers to the odd-numbered questions, and the full answer key is available only in the TEACH Instructor Resources. It is very important that you first complete the questions and then check your answers. The skill of medical coding can be acquired only through practice and by learning from mistakes that we all make along the way. It is from the understanding of why a service or diagnosis is coded in a certain way that you will develop a strong foundation that will serve you well throughout your coding career. Always take the time to read each code description fully, all notes connected with the code, and any applicable guidelines.

It is our sincere hope that you find the material presented in the *Workbook* challenging, enlightening, and worth your time and effort. Do your very best, and it will show in the quality of your work.

Carol J. Buck, MS
Jackie L. Koesterman, CPC

Some of the CPT code descriptions for physician services include physician extender services. Physician extenders, such as nurse practitioners, physician assistants, and nurse anesthetists, etc., provide medical services typically performed by a physician. Within this educational material the term "physician" may include "and other qualified health care professionals" depending on the code. Refer to the official CPT® code descriptions and guidelines to determine codes that are appropriate to report services provided by non-physician practitioners.

Contents

CHAPTER 1

Reimbursement, HIPAA, and Compliance

http://evolve.elsevier.com/Buck/step

THEORY

Without the use of reference material, answer the following:

1. What two groups of persons were added to those eligible for Medicare benefits after the initial establishment of the Medicare program?

   a. ______________________________

   b. ______________________________

2. To what government organization did the Secretary of the Department of Health and Human Services delegate the responsibility for administering the Medicare program?

   ____

3. What government organization handles the funds for the Medicare program?

   ____

4. There are three items that Medicare beneficiaries are responsible for paying before Medicare will begin to pay for services. What are these three items? ______________, ______________, and ______________

5. Medicare publishes the Medicare fee schedule and usually pays what percentage of the amounts indicated for services? ______________

6. The three components of work, overhead (practice expense), and malpractice are part of an RVU. What do the initials RVU stand for?

   ____

Odd-numbered answers are located in Appendix B.

7. According to the filing guidelines, providers must file claims for their Medicare patients within __________ months of the date of service.

8. What editions of the *Federal Register* would the outpatient facilities be interested in?

    ________________ and ________________

9. Under what act was a major change in Medicare in 1989 made possible?

    ____

10. Can a physician charge a patient to complete a Medicare form?

    ____

11. Individuals covered under Medicare are termed ________________.

12. The ________________ ________________ ________________ do the paperwork for Medicare and are usually insurance companies that have bid for a contract with CMS to handle the Medicare program for a specific area.

13. Medicare Part C is also known as ______________________________.

14. HIPAA stands for ____

    ____.

15. The most major change to the health care industry as a result of HIPAA was as a result of what portion of the act? ________________________

    ____

16. The transfer of electronic documentation is accomplished through the use of ________________ ________________ Interchange technology.

17. The number that is assigned to all providers as a result of HIPAA:

    ________________ ________________ Identification

18. Under the Relative Value Unit system, ________________ values are assigned to each service and are determined on the basis of the resources necessary to the physician's performance of the service.

19. The ________________ charge historically was specific for each physician, but in 1993, the charge for a service was the same for all physicians within a locality, regardless of the specialty.

Odd-numbered answers are located in Appendix B.

20. For co-surgeons, Medicare pays the lesser of the actual charge or

    __________% of the global fee, dividing the payment equally between the two surgeons.

21. Specific regulations for Medicare are contained in the

    ________________ ________________ Manual.

22. Within an HMO, there is usually an individual who has been assigned to monitor the services provided to the patient both inside the facility and outside the facility. This person is known as the

    ________________.

23. In this model of HMO, the HMO directly employs the physicians.

    ________________ Model

24. In this model of HMO, the HMO contracts with the physician to provide the service at a set fee. These organizations are known as

    ________________ ________________ Associations.

25. An all-inclusive care program for the elderly that provides a comprehensive package of services that permits the client to continue

    to live at home is known as ________________ for

    ________________-________________ Care for the Elderly (PACE).

Odd-numbered answers are located in Appendix B.

CHAPTER 2

An Overview of ICD-10-CM

http://evolve.elsevier.com/Buck/step

THEORY

Answer the following questions about the Overview of ICD-10-CM:

1. The CM in ICD-10-CM stands for "Clinical Modification."

   True False

2. The ICD-10-CM was designed for classification of patient morbidity and mortality.

   True False

3. ICD-10 is widely used in Europe.

   True False

4. The National Center for Health Statistics is responsible for the disease classification system in the United States.

   True False

5. The 10th revision of the International Classification of Diseases (ICD-10) was issued in 1989 by the World Health Organization.

   True False

6. The I-10 Index presents main terms in bold type.

   True False

7. The I-10 contains 20 chapters.

   True False

Odd-numbered answers are located in Appendix B.

8. All I-10 codes start with a letter and can have as many as 7 characters.

   True   False

9. The subterms in the Index modify the main term and are called essential modifiers.

   True   False

10. In the Tabular List, italicized type is used to identify codes not sequenced as first-listed diagnosis.

    True   False

11. Bold type is used throughout the entire Tabular List.

    True   False

12. There are two tables located within the Index to Diseases and Injuries, hypertension and neoplasm.

    True   False

13. NOS (not otherwise specified) is the equivalent of "unspecified."

    True   False

14. NEC is used when the I-10 code does not have codes that provide greater specificity.

    True   False

Identify the format of the chapters in the ICD-10-CM, Tabular List, in the proper sequence, from first to last:

15. ________________	a. subcategory
16. ________________	b. chapter
17. ________________	c. subclassification
18. ________________	d. section
19. ________________	e. category

Odd-numbered answers are located in Appendix B.

PRACTICAL

20. What does the Excludes1 note state under category code C50?

____

____

21. What does the Includes note state under category code I72?

____

____

22. Would category code H36 be sequenced as the first-listed diagnosis?

____

____

Using ICD-10-CM, Tabular List, locate the first pages of Chapter 9 and answer the following questions about the chapter:

23. The name of the chapter: ______________________________

____

24. The name of the first section: ______________________________

____

25. The description of the second category: ______________________________

____

26. The description of the first subcategory: ______________________________

____

27. What Excludes1 note applies to the first subcategory? ______________

____

Odd-numbered answers are located in Appendix B.

Underline the main terms to be located in the Alphabetic Index in the following diagnostic statements:

28. Chronic pancreatitis
29. Anus abscess
30. Acute cholecystitis
31. Abdominal pain
32. Neonatal mastitis
33. Head mass
34. Idiopathic hypotension
35. Nutritional dwarfism
36. Liver disorder
37. Chronic fatigue
38. Sleep-related leg cramp
39. Positive skin test
40. Tight chest

Odd-numbered answers are located in Appendix B.

ICD-10-CM Outpatient Coding and Reporting Guidelines

http://evolve.elsevier.com/Buck/step

THEORY

Using a current copy of the ICD-10-CM Guidelines for Coding and Reporting for Outpatient Services, *answer the following questions:*

1. Section IV Diagnostic Coding and Reporting Guidelines for Outpatient Services take precedence over the general and disease-specific guidelines.

   True False

2. Always begin the search for the correct code assignment in the Alphabetic Index.

   True False

3. When a patient presents for outpatient surgery and the surgery is canceled, report the reason why the surgery was canceled as the first-listed diagnosis.

   True False

4. The codes from A00 through Z99 are always reported as first-listed diagnoses.

   True False

5. When a final diagnosis has not been established by the provider, it is acceptable to report codes for the presenting signs and symptoms.

   True False

6. External Cause codes are located in the Alphabetic Index for Diseases under External Causes.

   True False

Odd-numbered answers are located in Appendix B.

7. Report all conditions that coexist, even if they are not addressed or do not affect management/treatment during that encounter.

   True False

8. For patients receiving diagnostic services only during an encounter/visit, sequence first the reason for the encounter/visit indicated in the medical record.

   True False

9. A patient with primary lung cancer with metastasis to the spine presents for radiation treatment of the spine. The first-listed diagnosis reported is the primary lung cancer.

   True False

10. For patients receiving preoperative evaluations, sequence first a code from the subcategory Z01.81, Encounter for preprocedural examinations, followed by findings related to the preoperative evaluation.

    True False

11. Routine prenatal outpatient visits for high-risk patients are reported with a first-listed diagnosis from category O09, Supervision of high-risk pregnancy.

    True False

12. Z codes may be reported as a principal diagnosis in the hospital setting.

    True False

13. Heart transplant status code Z94.1 should not be reported with a code from subcategory T86.2, Complications of heart transplant.

    True False

14. The External Cause codes can be reported as a first-listed diagnosis.

    True False

15. When a patient is admitted to observation for a complication following outpatient surgery, report the complication as the first-listed diagnosis.

    True False

Odd-numbered answers are located in Appendix B.

PRACTICAL

Assign ICD-10-CM first-listed diagnosis followed by additional diagnoses if appropriate:

16. Established 50-year-old patient with end-stage renal disease, currently receiving dialysis, is seen for acute left upper quadrant pain.

    First-listed Diagnosis: ______________________

    ICD-10-CM Code: __________

    Other Diagnosis: ______________________

    ICD-10-CM Code: __________

    Other Diagnosis: ______________________

    ICD-10-CM Code: __________

17. Established patient with complaints of shortness of breath. Upon examination, the physician determined she needed more aggressive treatment for her current congestive heart failure.

    First-listed Diagnosis: ______________________

    ICD-10-CM Code: __________

18. Patient is seen for unstable angina. He has a history of arteriosclerotic coronary artery disease.

    First-listed Diagnosis: ______________________

    ICD-10-CM Code: __________

19. Patient is seen for follow-up for hypertension. He has end-stage renal disease.

    First-listed Diagnosis: ______________________

    ICD-10-CM Code: __________

    Other Diagnosis: ______________________

    ICD-10-CM Code: __________

Odd-numbered answers are located in Appendix B.

20. Encounter for chemotherapy for prostate cancer.

    First-listed Diagnosis: ______________________________

    ICD-10-CM Code: ______________

    Other Diagnosis: ______________________________

    ICD-10-CM Code: ______________

21. Patient with chronic obstructive pulmonary disease (COPD) is seen for an acute lower respiratory tract infection.

    First-listed Diagnosis: ______________________________

    ICD-10-CM Code: ______________

22. Patient was scheduled for outpatient surgery for right inguinal hernia repair; however, he has a fever and a URI, and the procedure is canceled.

    First-listed Diagnosis: ______________________________

    ICD-10-CM Code: ______________

    Other Diagnosis: ______________________________

    ICD-10-CM Code: ______________

    Other Diagnosis: ______________________________

    ICD-10-CM Code: ______________

23. An otherwise healthy patient is seen in the clinic for exposure to tuberculosis.

    First-listed Diagnosis: ______________________________

    ICD-10-CM Code: ______________

24. Patient presents for an outpatient chest x-ray, due to chest pain with breathing. Finding later indicated: normal x-ray.

    First-listed Diagnosis: ______________________________

    ICD-10-CM Code: ______________

Odd-numbered answers are located in Appendix B.

25. Patient, with known cardiovascular disease, is seen for a follow-up visit to discuss results of a cardiac perfusion study (cardiovascular function study), which was abnormal.

    First-listed Diagnosis: ____________________

    ICD-10-CM Code: ____________

    Other Diagnosis: ____________________

    ICD-10-CM Code: ____________

26. Following outpatient surgery for a right bunionectomy for hallux valgus, the patient was admitted to observation due to an exacerbation of her asthma postprocedure.

    First-listed Diagnosis: ____________________

    ICD-10-CM Code: ____________

    Other Diagnosis: ____________________

    ICD-10-CM Code: ____________

27. A patient presents with a contusion to the left cheek that resulted from a fistfight, initial encounter.

    First-listed Diagnosis: ____________________

    ICD-10-CM Code: ____________

    Other Diagnosis: ____________________

    ICD-10-CM Code: ____________

28. Patient presents with a fracture of the right femur shaft due to a fall from her horse while riding, initial encounter.

    First-listed Diagnosis: ____________________

    ICD-10-CM Code: ____________

    Other Diagnosis: ____________________

    ICD-10-CM Code: ____________

    Other Diagnosis: ____________________

    ICD-10-CM Code: ____________

Odd-numbered answers are located in Appendix B.

29. Encounter for insulin pump titration.

    First-listed Diagnosis: ______________________

    ICD-10-CM Code: __________

30. Patient in her second trimester is seen for a regular prenatal visit. She has a history of ectopic pregnancy.

    First-listed Diagnosis: ______________________

    ICD-10-CM Code: __________

31. Twin born via vaginal delivery, liveborn in the hospital.

    First-listed Diagnosis: ______________________

    ICD-10-CM Code: __________

32. Encounter for change of nephrostomy tube.

    First-listed Diagnosis: ______________________

    ICD-10-CM Code: __________

33. A patient was seen for an abrasion of the left upper arm, initial encounter.

    First-listed Diagnosis: ______________________

    ICD-10-CM Code: __________

34. Established patient is seen for hypertension, and a prescription is refilled for psoriasis.

    First-listed Diagnosis: ______________________

    ICD-10-CM Code: __________

    Other Diagnosis: ______________________

    ICD-10-CM Code: __________

35. A patient who smokes 2 packs of cigarettes per day and suffers with chronic pulmonary disease is seen in follow-up for acute bronchitis.

    First-listed Diagnosis: ______________________

    ICD-10-CM Code: __________

    Other Diagnoses: __________, __________

    ICD-10-CM Code: __________, __________

Odd-numbered answers are located in Appendix B.

Using ICD-10-CM

http://evolve.elsevier.com/Buck/step

THEORY

Without the use of reference material, answer the following:

1. An example of a late effect is hemorrhage after a surgery requiring a return to the operating room.

   True False

2. You may report a code from the Index without verifying in the Tabular when there is no indication that the code requires additional characters.

   True False

3. If a patient has a confirmed diagnosis, the signs and symptoms related to that condition should also be reported.

   True False

4. If the same condition is described as both acute and chronic, and separate subentries exist in the Alphabetic Index at the same indentation level, report both codes and sequence the acute code first.

   True False

5. A dash (-) at the end of an Index entry indicates that an additional character or characters is/are required.

   True False

6. Cholelithiasis with chronic cholecystitis without obstruction (K80.10) is an example of a dual code.

   True False

7. A code is invalid if it has not been reported to the full number of characters available, including the 7th character, if applicable.

   True False

Odd-numbered answers are located in Appendix B.

8. In most cases the manifestation codes will have in the code title "in diseases classified elsewhere."

   True False

9. A late effect usually occurs within 1 month of the illness or injury.

   True False

10. In diabetic retinopathy, the retinopathy is the etiology and the diabetes is the manifestation.

    True False

11. In the outpatient setting, it is correct to report a "probable" condition as if it exists, such as probable appendicitis as appendicitis.

    True False

12. When sequencing codes for residuals and late effects, the late effect code is sequenced first followed by a code describing the residual condition.

    True False

13. Section II of the *ICD-10-CM Official Guidelines for Coding and Reporting* includes instructions on outpatient coding and reporting.

    True False

14. Diagnosis codes are always reported to the highest number of characters available.

    True False

15. The cooperating parties for the development and approval of the *Official Guidelines for Coding and Reporting* are CMS, AMA, and NCHS.

    True False

16. List two common symptoms associated with acute myocardial infarction.

    ____________________ ____________________

17. List two common symptoms associated with gastroesophageal reflux.

    ____________________ ____________________

18. List two common symptoms associated with seasonal allergies.

    ____________________ ____________________

Odd-numbered answers are located in Appendix B.

19. List two symptoms of a broken nose.

_______________ _______________

Identify the Residual and Cause of the following diagnoses:

20. Acute renal failure due to previous viral encephalitis.

Residual: ____________________

Cause: ____________________

21. Constrictive pericarditis due to old tuberculosis infection.

Residual: ____________________

Cause: ____________________

22. Hemiplegia/hemiparesis affecting right dominant side due to cerebrovascular accident 4 months ago.

Residual: ____________________

Cause: ____________________

PRACTICAL

Using the ICD-10-CM, code the following:

23. Acute and chronic sinusitis.

ICD-10-CM Codes: ____________, ____________

24. Acute and chronic tonsillitis.

ICD-10-CM Codes: ____________, ____________

25. Pneumoconiosis due to lime dust.

ICD-10-CM Code: ____________

26. Neuritis due to herniation of nucleus pulposus.

ICD-10-CM Codes: ____________, ____________

27. Pneumonitis due to *Hemophilus influenzae.*

ICD-10-CM Code: ____________

28. Patient has unstable angina.

ICD-10-CM Code: ____________

Odd-numbered answers are located in Appendix B.

29. Threatened shock, patient is hypotensive.

    ICD-10-CM Code: ______________

30. Adult osteomalacia due to malnutrition.

    ICD-10-CM Code: ______________

31. Pancreatitis, acute and chronic.

    ICD-10-CM Codes: ______________, ______________

32. Systemic lupus erythematosus causing endocarditis.

    ICD-10-CM Code: ______________

33. Vitamin D–resistant rickets.

    ICD-10-CM Codes: ______________, ______________

34. Febrile complex convulsions with status epilepticus.

    ICD-10-CM Code: ______________

35. Ascites in alcoholic hepatitis, alcohol use unspecified.

    ICD-10-CM Codes: ______________, ______________

Odd-numbered answers are located in Appendix B.

CHAPTER 5

Chapter-Specific Guidelines (ICD-10-CM Chapters 1-10)

http://evolve.elsevier.com/Buck/step

THEORY

Answer the following questions about the overview of ICD-10-CM:

1. Combination coding is when one code fully describes the conditions and/or manifestations.

   True False

2. For hemiplegia and hemiparesis and other paralytic syndromes, report the right side as dominant if the documentation does not specify which side is dominant.

   True False

3. When reporting an infection, other than *Staphylococcus aureus*, that is antibiotic resistant, report the infection first followed by a code from category Z16, Infection with drug resistant microorganisms.

   True False

4. Diabetes mellitus codes are combination codes that include the type of diabetes as well as the body system involved and complications affecting the body system.

   True False

5. Methicillin-resistant *Streptococcus aureus* is also referred to as MRSA.

   True False

6. For reporting purposes, urosepsis is not considered sepsis.

   True False

7. If the medical documentation indicates the patient has two conditions that are both included in one diagnosis code, report that diagnosis code only once.

   True False

Odd-numbered answers are located in Appendix B.

8. Multiple coding is when it takes more than one code to fully describe the condition, circumstance, or manifestation.

   True False

9. When the histological type of neoplasm is documented, reference the Alphabetic Index first rather than going immediately to the Neoplasm Table.

   True False

10. SIRS is the diagnosis when all of the following are diagnosed: hypothermia or fever, tachycardia, tachypnea, increased or decreased white blood count.

    True False

11. Viral hepatitis codes are divided based on the type of hepatitis and if the condition is with or without hepatic coma.

    True False

12. If a patient is admitted with pneumonia and while hospitalized develops severe sepsis, you would report the pneumonia first, followed by the severe sepsis.

    True False

13. When an encounter is for treatment of anemia due to a malignancy, the first-listed diagnosis would be the malignancy, followed by the anemia.

    True False

14. An "Uncertain" neoplasm is one that is not clearly benign or malignant.

    True False

15. Septic shock is considered organ failure.

    True False

16. Hepatitis A was formerly known as infectious or epidemic hepatitis.

    True False

17. Epiphora is a blockage of the lacrimal passage.

    True False

Odd-numbered answers are located in Appendix B.

18. When reporting hypertensive chronic kidney disease, an additional code to report the type of chronic kidney disease is not required.

    True False

19. A Q-wave or transmural myocardial infarction, also known as STEMI, is the most severe type of infarction.

    True False

20. Only confirmed cases of COVID-19 can be reported.

    True False

PRACTICAL

Using the ICD-10-CM, code the following:

21. Acute renal failure and acute respiratory failure due to sepsis.

    ICD-10-CM Codes: ______________, ______________,

    ______________, ______________

22. A patient with early onset Alzheimer's progresses to combative behavior.

    ICD-10-CM Codes: ______________, ______________

23. Patient with known hepatitis B seen in the clinic complaining of joint pain, loss of appetite, nausea and vomiting, and weakness and fatigue. He is admitted to the hospital for severe dehydration.

    ICD-10-CM Codes: ______________, ______________

24. An obstetric patient in her third trimester of pregnancy is admitted for *Pneumocystis carinii* pneumonia due to AIDS.

    ICD-10-CM Codes: ______________, ______________, ______________

25. Lung abscess due to MRSA (methicillin-resistant *Staphylococcus aureus*).

    ICD-10-CM Codes: ______________, ______________

26. Patient presents for HIV screening; patient is asymptomatic.

    ICD-10-CM Code: ______________

27. Patient presents for follow-up exam following reconstructive surgery to repair hypospadias.

    ICD-10-CM Codes: ______________, ______________

Odd-numbered answers are located in Appendix B.

28. Initial encounter for a 45-year-old woman receiving her first cycle of chemotherapy for pancreatic cancer is seen in the emergency room for severe nausea and vomiting due to the chemotherapy. She is admitted for dehydration.

    ICD-10-CM Codes: ______________, ______________, ______________

29. Patient seen in an outpatient clinic with ascites due to disseminated malignant neoplasm.

    ICD-10-CM Codes: ______________, ______________

30. Hypertensive heart disease, with congestive heart failure.

    ICD-10-CM Codes: ______________, ______________

31. Patient seen for cellulitis of left lower leg. He is a type 2 diabetic controlled with oral medications. The cellulitis has elevated his blood glucose, and the physician elects to treat with sliding-scale insulin regimen.

    ICD-10-CM Codes: ______________, ______________

32. A 62-year-old man admitted to the hospital from the emergency room diagnosed with a transmural Q wave infarction. He has ASHD and had a pacemaker placed 5 years ago.

    ICD-10-CM Codes: ______________, ______________, ______________

33. Patient seen in consult by a high-risk obstetrician. She is 2 months pregnant and was diagnosed with a malignant neoplasm of the left breast.

    ICD-10-CM Codes: ______________, ______________

34. Initial encounter for a patient with sepsis due to a blood transfusion. He has hemophilia.

    ICD-10-CM Codes: ______________, ______________, ______________

35. Patient with anemia due to prostate cancer.

    ICD-10-CM Codes: ______________, ______________

36. Patient is admitted for chemotherapy for primary liver cancer.

    ICD-10-CM Codes: ______________, ______________

37. Patient admitted to hospital for bowel obstruction. This patient is also hypertensive with chronic kidney disease, stage 5.

    ICD-10-CM Codes: ______________, ______________, ______________

Odd-numbered answers are located in Appendix B.

38. Patient is following up at her oncologist's office for treatment options of metastatic cancer to right axillary lymph nodes. She has a history of right upper-outer quadrant breast cancer, still receiving treatment.

    ICD-10-CM Codes: ______________, ______________

39. Patient underwent a biopsy of the brain. The pathology report indicates secondary cancer from the primary site of the breast. The patient had a left mastectomy 5 years ago and currently receives no treatment for breast cancer.

    ICD-10-CM Codes: ______________, ______________, ______________

40. Patient underwent fulguration of malignant bladder tumors.

    ICD-10-CM Code: ______________

41. Patient with polycythemia vera presented to an outpatient clinic for a phlebotomy.

    ICD-10-CM Code: ______________

42. A 45-year-old man seen in the office with suspected contact with COVID-19.

    ICD-10-CM Code: ______________

43. Initial encounter for failure of insulin pump causing an overdose of insulin and hypoglycemic (level 3) coma. The patient is a type 1 diabetic.

    ICD-10-CM Codes: ______________, ______________, ______________, ______________

44. Patient diagnosed with dementia with Lewy bodies.

    ICD-10-CM Codes: ______________, ______________

45. Patient admitted to the hospital for resection of a malignant lung tumor from the right upper lobe.

    ICD-10-CM Code: ______________

46. A man arrested for disorderly conduct is brought to the emergency room. He is a known alcoholic-dependent patient. Alcohol blood level indicates intoxication.

    ICD-10-CM Code: ______________

47. Patient with chest pain is admitted to the hospital. He is diagnosed with acute Q wave myocardial infarction.

    ICD-10-CM Code: ______________

Odd-numbered answers are located in Appendix B.

48. Initial encounter for cardiac arrest due to cocaine dependence.

    ICD-10-CM Codes: _______________, _______________, _______________

49. Schizophrenic with disorderly conduct noncompliant with his medications.

    ICD-10-CM Codes: _______________, _______________, _______________

50. Delirium tremors due to withdrawal from cocaine dependence.

    ICD-10-CM Code: _______________

51. Meningitis caused by measles.

    ICD-10-CM Code: _______________

52. Mononeuropathy of right lower limb due to diabetes, type 2.

    ICD-10-CM Code: _______________

53. Polyneuropathy and arthritis due to syphilis.

    ICD-10-CM Codes: _______________, _______________

54. Streptococcal arthritis.

    ICD-10-CM Codes: _______________, _______________

55. Patient admitted with left hemiplegia and cerebral palsy for evaluation for possible baclofen pump to treat spasticity.

    ICD-10-CM Code: _______________

User to decide number of codes necessary to correctly answer the question.

56. Bilateral sensorineural deafness following bacterial meningitis.

    ICD-10-CM Code(s): _______________

57. Ménière's disease.

    ICD-10-CM Code(s): _______________

58. Right carotid stenosis causing a cerebral infarct.

    ICD-10-CM Code(s): _______________

User to decide number of codes necessary to correctly answer the question.

Odd-numbered answers are located in Appendix B.

59. Acute pulmonary edema due to left heart failure. Patient now intubated and on a respirator.

    ICD-10-CM Code(s): ______________

REPORTS

In Appendix A of this workbook you will find a section titled Reports, which contains original reports. Read the report indicated below and supply the appropriate ICD-10-CM codes on the following lines:

60. Report 7

    ICD-10-CM Code(s): ______________

61. Report 9

    ICD-10-CM Code(s): ______________

62. Report 19

    ICD-10-CM Code(s): ______________

63. Report 20

    ICD-10-CM Code(s): ______________

64. Report 34

    ICD-10-CM Code(s): ______________

65. Report 39

    ICD-10-CM Code(s): ______________

66. Report 40

    ICD-10-CM Code(s): ______________

67. Report 42

    ICD-10-CM Code(s): ______________

68. Report 44

    ICD-10-CM Code(s): ______________

69. Report 90

    ICD-10-CM Code(s): ______________

User to decide number of codes necessary to correctly answer the question.

Odd-numbered answers are located in Appendix B.

Chapter-Specific Guidelines (ICD-10-CM Chapters 11-14)

http://evolve.elsevier.com/Buck/step

THEORY

Answer the following questions about the ICD-10-CM Guidelines for Coding and Reporting for Outpatient Services:

1. Includes and Excludes notes are only listed in the Tabular of the ICD-10-CM.

   True False

2. Chapter 12, Diseases of the Skin and Subcutaneous Tissue, describes diseases or conditions of the integumentary and musculoskeletal systems.

   True False

3. In the ICD-10-CM, pressure ulcers are graded and reported based on the depth of the ulcer.

   True False

4. Code range M00-M02 reports infectious arthropathies due to infections that are direct or indirect.

   True False

5. Chapter 13 of the *ICD-10-CM Guidelines for Coding and Reporting* indicates the 7th character D is assigned as long as the patient is receiving active treatment for a fracture.

   True False

6. The two types of indirect infections are reactive and postinfective arthropathy.

   True False

7. To report a hemorrhage, active bleeding must be present.

   True False

Odd-numbered answers are located in Appendix B.

8. The categories in Chapter 11, Diseases of the Digestive System, begin when food enters the mouth and continue to when it leaves the body through the anus.

   True False

9. Conditions affecting the nails, sweat glands, and hair are located in Chapter 12.

   True False

10. The "Code first" note directs the coder to report first the underlying disease.

    True False

PRACTICAL

Using the ICD-10-CM, code the following:

11. Patient is seen for erosion of the teeth due to diet.

    ICD-10-CM Code: ______________

12. Abscess of the salivary glands.

    ICD-10-CM Code: ______________

13. Hemorrhage of the fallopian tube.

    ICD-10-CM Code: ______________

14. Chronic prostatitis with hematuria.

    ICD-10-CM Codes: ______________, ______________

15. Cellulitis of female external genital organs.

    ICD-10-CM Code: ______________

16. Stiffness of the right wrist.

    ICD-10-CM Code: ______________

17. Congenital paraphimosis.

    ICD-10-CM Code: ______________

18. Submandibular abscess.

    ICD-10-CM Code: ______________

Odd-numbered answers are located in Appendix B.

19. Secondary amenorrhea.

    ICD-10-CM Code: ______________

20. Ligament disorder of the right foot joint.

    ICD-10-CM Code: ______________

21. Patient suffers a nontraumatic hematoma of the soft tissue.

    ICD-10-CM Code: ______________

22. Old sacroiliac joint lesion.

    ICD-10-CM Code: ______________

23. Inflammatory polyps of colon with intestinal obstruction.

    ICD-10-CM Code: ______________

24. Hypertrophic scar.

    ICD-10-CM Code: ______________

25. Chronic ulcer of the right thigh, non-pressure, with exposure of fat layer.

    ICD-10-CM Code: ______________

26. Acute recurrent sialoadenitis.

    ICD-10-CM Code: ______________

27. Unilateral internal inguinal hernia with gangrene, recurrent.

    ICD-10-CM Code: ______________

28. Acute osteomyelitis of the right radius and ulna.

    ICD-10-CM Code: ______________

29. Chronic nephritic syndrome with focal glomerulonephritis.

    ICD-10-CM Code: ______________

30. Patient with end-stage renal disease, currently on hemodialysis.

    ICD-10-CM Codes: ______________, ______________

31. Infected pilonidal fistula with abscess.

    ICD-10-CM Code: ______________

Odd-numbered answers are located in Appendix B.

32. Cradle cap.

    ICD-10-CM Code: ______________

33. Interstitial myositis of the left lower leg.

    ICD-10-CM Code: ______________

34. Abnormal uterine bleeding unrelated to menstrual cycle.

    ICD-10-CM Code: ______________

35. Systemic lupus erythematosus with lung involvement.

    ICD-10-CM Code: ______________

36. *Staphylococcus aureus* arthritis of right carpal bones.

    ICD-10-CM Codes: ______________, ______________

37. Streptococcal group B arthritis of the metacarpus and phalanges, left hand.

    ICD-10-CM Codes: ______________, ______________

38. Endometriosis of the left ovary and fallopian tube.

    ICD-10-CM Codes: ______________, ______________

39. Patient is seen for a foreign body granuloma of the soft tissue, right upper arm.

    ICD-10-CM Code: ______________

User to decide number of codes necessary to correctly answer the question.

40. Localized acute appendicitis with peritonitis with perforation of appendix.

    ICD-10-CM Code(s): ______________

41. Chronic abscess of the areola of the right breast, unrelated to the puerperium.

    ICD-10-CM Code(s): ______________

42. Cyst of the Bartholin's gland.

    ICD-10-CM Code(s): ______________

User to decide number of codes necessary to correctly answer the question.

Odd-numbered answers are located in Appendix B.

REPORTS

In Appendix A of this workbook you will find a section titled Reports, which contains original reports. Read the reports indicated below and supply the appropriate ICD-10-CM codes on the following lines:

43. Report 6 ICD-10-CM Code(s): ___________
44. Report 8 ICD-10-CM Code(s): ___________
45. Report 10 ICD-10-CM Code(s): ___________
46. Report 11 ICD-10-CM Code(s): ___________
47. Report 12 ICD-10-CM Code(s): ___________
48. Report 13 ICD-10-CM Code(s): ___________
49. Report 14 ICD-10-CM Code(s): ___________
50. Report 15 ICD-10-CM Code(s): ___________
51. Report 31 ICD-10-CM Code(s): ___________
52. Report 32 ICD-10-CM Code(s): ___________
53. Report 33 ICD-10-CM Code(s): ___________
54. Report 35 ICD-10-CM Code(s): ___________
55. Report 38 ICD-10-CM Code(s): ___________
56. Report 41 ICD-10-CM Code(s): ___________
57. Report 43 ICD-10-CM Code(s): ___________
58. Report 91 ICD-10-CM Code(s): ___________
59. Report 92 ICD-10-CM Code(s): ___________
60. Report 93 ICD-10-CM Code(s): ___________

User to decide number of codes necessary to correctly answer the question.

Odd-numbered answers are located in Appendix B.

CHAPTER 7

Chapter-Specific Guidelines (ICD-10-CM Chapters 15-22)

http://evolve.elsevier.com/Buck/step

THEORY

Answer the following questions about the ICD-10-CM Guidelines for Coding and Reporting for Outpatient Services:

1. Codes from Chapter 17, Congenital Anomalies, can be reported any time during a person's life, as appropriate.

   True False

2. Chapter 15 codes are never reported on the mother's record.

   True False

3. The first-listed diagnosis for a routine outpatient prenatal visit is a code from category Z34, Encounter for supervision of normal pregnancy.

   True False

4. The outcome of delivery is reported only on the newborn's record.

   True False

5. The third trimester is considered 28 weeks 0 days from the first day of LMP until delivery occurs.

   True False

6. A hydatidiform mole is a tumor that only forms in the uterus.

   True False

7. When there is an encounter for a complication and no delivery occurred, report the complication as the first-listed condition.

   True False

Odd-numbered answers are located in Appendix B.

8. When coding the birth episode in a newborn record, assign a code from Category Z38, Liveborn infants, according to place of birth and type of delivery, as the first-listed diagnosis.

   True False

9. ICD-10-CM contains combination codes that identify only definitive diagnoses.

   True False

10. The aftercare Z codes should not be reported for aftercare of injuries.

    True False

11. Multiple fractures are sequenced in accordance to the location of the fracture.

    True False

12. Corrosions are a result of a chemical contact and are classified by the depth, extent, and corrosive agent.

    True False

13. You would assign an adverse effect code when a drug that was correctly prescribed and administered resulted in an adverse effect.

    True False

14. When reporting multiple burns, sequence first the code that reports the highest degree of burn.

    True False

15. Functional quadriplegia is the lack of ability to use one's limbs and is not associated with neurologic deficit or injury.

    True False

With the use of reference material, answer the following:

16. When assigning one of the O10 codes that include hypertensive heart disease or hypertensive chronic kidney disease, it is necessary to add a

    ________________ code from the appropriate hypertension category to specify the type of heart failure or chronic kidney disease.

17. A(n) ________________ is an abnormality of a structure or organ.

Odd-numbered answers are located in Appendix B.

18. A(n) ________________ is defined as objective evidence of a disease that can be observed by the physician. A(n) ________________ is a subjective observation reported by the patient.

19. One method to locate abnormal findings in the Index of the I-10 is to reference the main term ________________ and subterm by specific test.

20. Most categories in Chapter 19 of the ICD-10 have 7th character extensions. Most categories in this chapter have three extensions (with the exception of fractures): A, initial encounter, D, subsequent encounter, and ________________, sequela.

21. A patient presents with second- and third-degree burns of the arm. What is the only degree of burn reported?

    ____

22. According to the guidelines on poisoning, ________________ refers to taking less of a medication than is prescribed by a provider.

23. Codes from Chapter ________________ of the Tabular of the I-10 report symptoms, signs, and abnormal clinical and laboratory findings.

24. Chapter ________________ of the Tabular of the I-10 is probably the most difficult chapter from which to report diagnoses due to the complexity of coding.

25. According to the guidelines, when sequencing multiple fractures, sequence in accordance with the ________________ of the fracture.

PRACTICAL

Using the ICD-10-CM, code the following:

26. Induced abortion complicated by endometritis.

    ICD-10-CM Code: ____________

27. Abrasion of the left upper arm, initial encounter.

    ICD-10-CM Code: ____________

28. Hepatomegaly.

    ICD-10-CM Code: ____________

Odd-numbered answers are located in Appendix B.

29. Anaphylactic shock, initial encounter.

    ICD-10-CM Code: ______________

30. Failure to gain weight, child.

    ICD-10-CM Code: ______________

31. Pelvic peritonitis following ectopic pregnancy without intrauterine pregnancy.

    ICD-10-CM Codes: ______________, ______________

32. Initial encounter of a patient transported to emergency department. Patient died from cardiac arrest due to an accidental overdose from heroin abuse.

    ICD-10-CM Codes: ______________, ______________, ______________

33. Concealed penis.

    ICD-10-CM Code: ______________

34. Crush syndrome, subsequent encounter.

    ICD-10-CM Code: ______________

35. A 24-year-old woman at 32 weeks' gestation has hypotension.

    ICD-10-CM Codes: ______________, ______________

36. Newborn with cellulitis of the navel with mild hemorrhage.

    ICD-10-CM Code: ______________

37. Inability to swallow.

    ICD-10-CM Code: ______________

38. Absence of bowel sounds.

    ICD-10-CM Code: ______________

39. Sprain, left ankle, initial encounter.

    ICD-10-CM Code: ______________

40. Newborn with primary obstructive sleep apnea.

    ICD-10-CM Code: ______________

41. First- and second-degree burn, right hand, subsequent encounter.

    ICD-10-CM Code: ______________

Odd-numbered answers are located in Appendix B.

42. Partial traumatic amputation of the left index finger, initial encounter.

    ICD-10-CM Code: ______________

43. Patient with persistent proteinuria.

    ICD-10-CM Code: ______________

44. Accidental overdose of ibuprofen [NSAID], initial encounter.

    ICD-10-CM Code: ______________

45. Hematoma of the nose, subsequent encounter.

    ICD-10-CM Code: ______________

46. Newborn female delivered in the hospital by cesarean delivery.

    ICD-10-CM Code: ______________

47. Fragile X syndrome.

    ICD-10-CM Code: ______________

48. Anemia due to prematurity of infant.

    ICD-10-CM Code: ______________

49. A 26-year-old woman at 30 weeks' gestation with quadruplets.

    ICD-10-CM Codes: ______________, ______________

User to decide number of codes necessary to correctly answer the question.

50. Unexplained death, prior to entering health care facility.

    ICD-10-CM Code(s): ______________

51. Tremors due to accidental overdose of monoamine oxidase, initial encounter.

    ICD-10-CM Code(s): ______________

52. Nausea and vomiting.

    ICD-10-CM Code(s): ______________

User to decide number of codes necessary to correctly answer the question.

Odd-numbered answers are located in Appendix B.

53. Blister of the right wrist, initial encounter.

    ICD-10-CM Code(s): ______________

54. Acute gastritis with bleeding due to adverse effect of omeprazole, initial encounter.

    ICD-10-CM Code(s): ______________

55. Subsequent encounter for fracture, right clavicle, with delayed healing.

    ICD-10-CM Code(s): ______________

56. Positive occult blood in stools.

    ICD-10-CM Code(s): ______________

57. Adult with respiratory distress and extreme fatigue.

    ICD-10-CM Code(s): ______________

58. Vaginal pain.

    ICD-10-CM Code(s): ______________

REPORTS

In Appendix A of this workbook you will find a section titled Reports, which contains original reports. Read the reports indicated below and supply the appropriate ICD-10-CM codes on the following lines:

59. Report 28

    ICD-10-CM Code(s): ______________

60. Report 36

    ICD-10-CM Code(s): ______________

61. Report 40

    ICD-10-CM Code(s): ______________

62. Report 94

    ICD-10-CM Code(s): ______________

63. Report 95

    ICD-10-CM Code(s): ______________

User to decide number of codes necessary to correctly answer the question.

Odd-numbered answers are located in Appendix B.

CHAPTER 8

Introduction to CPT

http://evolve.elsevier.com/Buck/step

THEORY

Without the use of reference material, complete the following:

There are six index location methods presented in Chapter 8. List any four of the methods.

1. ______________________

2. ______________________

3. ______________________

4. ______________________

Match the appendix with the information it contains:

5. ____ Appendix E — a. Modifier -63 Information on Infants <4 kg

6. ____ Appendix F — b. Add-on Codes

7. ____ Appendix D — c. Product Pending FDA Approval

8. ____ Appendix K — d. Modifier -51 exempt

9. You would expect to find the CPT code 71045 in what section of the CPT manual?

____

10. What is the report called that a physician dictates to show that an unusual or rare procedure is performed?

____

11. What association publishes the CPT?

____

Odd-numbered answers are located in Appendix B.

12. When you see the symbol ▲ in front of a code, you know what about the code?

____

13. What type of code has the full code description? ____________

14. What type of code has only a portion of the code description?

____

15. What would providers enter on the insurance form to show payers which services or procedures were performed?

____________ and/or ____________

16. The use of a coding system allows you to communicate not only quickly, but also ____________.

17. The first edition of the CPT was published in what year? ____________

18. The updated CPT manual is available for purchase in what month?

____

19. A standard for communicating health care data, as represented in CPT, was necessary to address requirements of this 1996 act:

____

____________ and ____________ Act.

20. What does the symbol of a circle with a line through it (⊘) placed before a CPT code indicate about the code?

____

PRACTICAL

With the use of the CPT manual section Guidelines, identify the following unlisted codes:

Radiology

21. Clinical brachytherapy ____________

22. Therapeutic radiology clinical treatment planning ____________

23. Therapeutic radiology treatment management ____________

Odd-numbered answers are located in Appendix B.

Pathology and Laboratory

24. Surgical pathology procedure ___________________

25. Urinalysis procedure ___________________

Medicine

26. Allergy/clinical immunological service ___________________

27. Special dermatological service ___________________

28. Dialysis procedures, inpatient or outpatient ___________________

Odd-numbered answers are located in Appendix B.

CHAPTER 9

Introduction to the Level II National Codes (HCPCS)

http://evolve.elsevier.com/Buck/step

THEORY

Without the use of reference material, complete the following:

HCPCS is a collection of codes that may be provided to Medicare and Medicaid beneficiaries to represent these four items.

1. ______________________
2. ______________________
3. ______________________
4. ______________________
5. Level II codes (National Codes) are approved and maintained by this workgroup. ______________________
6. Level II National Modifiers are located in the introduction section of the HCPCS and also in what Appendix of CPT? ______________________
7. G codes are used to identify what type of procedures and services that would otherwise be reported with a CPT code, but no CPT code has been established?

   ____

8. Medicare and other federal payers do not recognize "S" codes; however, "S" codes may be useful for claims to what type of insurers?

   ____

Odd numbered answers are located in Appendix B.

List the temporary code letters for procedures or services that are not established by private payers or Medicaid.

9. ___________________________

10. ___________________________

11. ___________________________

12. HCPCS codes J9000-J9999 cover the cost of the chemotherapy drug. What is not included in payment for the reported J code?

____

13. Items billed before a signed and dated order has been received by the supplier must be submitted with this modifier.

____

14. This HCPCS modifier indicates a required Waiver of Liability was issued to the patient.

____

15. HCPCS codes that are used to identify services that would not be reported with a CPT code, such as drugs, biologicals, and types of medical equipment/services, which are not identified by Level II National codes.

____

Match the following administration methods for drugs:

16. _____ OTH — a. Subcutaneous

17. _____ IT — b. Inhalant solution

18. _____ IV — c. Various routes

19. _____ IM — d. Intrathecal

20. _____ SC — e. Intramuscular

21. _____ INH — f. Intravenous

22. _____ VAR — g. Other routes

Odd-numbered answers are located in Appendix B.

PRACTICAL

With the use of the HCPCS Level II manual section Index, identify the following codes:

23. Abatacept ____________________
24. Bacterial sensitivity study ____________________
25. Carbon filter ____________________
26. Cerumen, removal ____________________
27. Ear mold, not disposable ____________________
28. Paclitaxel, 1 mg ____________________
29. Wheelchair, narrowing device ____________________
30. Vaccine administration, influenza ____________________
31. Vaccine administration, pneumococcal ____________________
32. Walking boot, non-pneumatic, customized ____________________

Odd-numbered answers are located in Appendix B.

CHAPTER 10

Modifiers

http://evolve.elsevier.com/Buck/step

THEORY

Without the use of reference material, answer the following:

1. What appendix in the CPT manual contains a complete list of all modifiers?

   ____

2. What is the word that means assigning multiple codes when one code would do?

   ____

3. What is the term that describes the services provided to a patient by the physician before surgery?

   ____

4. What is another term for the time after the surgery that the physician provides services to the patient?

   ____

5. Do all third-party payers recognize all modifiers as listed in the CPT manual?

   ____

6. What is the term that describes two physicians working together in the completion of a procedure when each has the same level of responsibility?

   ____

Odd-numbered answers are located in Appendix B.

PRACTICAL

Using the CPT and ICD-10-CM manuals, indicate the modifiers and diagnoses that would be reported for the following:

7. A patient is admitted and has bilateral arthroscopy of the knees due to Baker's cysts.

   Modifier: ___________

   ICD-10-CM Codes: _______________, _______________

8. Ben Carter, surgical resident, assists Dr. Wells, chief cardiologist, in a coronary artery bypass procedure due to coronary arteriosclerosis of a native artery. What modifier would be submitted to report Ben's services in the teaching hospital?

   Modifier: ___________

   ICD-10-CM Code: _______________

9. Dr. Wells began surgery for right knee replacement due to severe osteoarthritis on an 86-year-old female with controlled hypertension. The patient was satisfactorily anesthetized, and the site opened to view. Shortly thereafter, the patient's blood pressure dropped significantly, and the physician was unable to stabilize the patient. The procedure was discontinued.

   Modifier: ___________

   ICD-10-CM Codes: _______________, _______________, _______________

10. The patient is a 10-month-old boy who fell while trying to walk across the kitchen floor at his home. He suffered an open wound to his bottom lip. Sutures are necessary, but due to the patient's age and excessive movement, general anesthesia is needed.

    Modifier: ___________

    ICD-10-CM Codes: Diagnosis: _______________

    External Cause W Code: _______________

    External Cause Y Code Place of Occurrence: _______________

11. A radiological examination of the gastrointestinal tract was ordered by a third-party payer for a confirmation of Crohn's disease (regional enteritis) of the large bowel. Crohn's was confirmed.

    Modifier: ___________

    ICD-10-CM Code: _______________

Odd-numbered answers are located in Appendix B.

12. Anesthesia provided by the ENT physician during a tympanoplasty for repair of a tympanic membrane perforation.

    Modifier: ___________

    ICD-10-CM Code: ______________

13. A patient is seen at the direction of Workers' Compensation for a complete physical examination for insurance certification.

    Modifier: ___________

    ICD-10-CM Code: ______________

14. The patient returns to the operating room by the same physician for removal of deep pins during the postoperative period due to complication (dislodgement) after an open repair of a humerus fracture.

    Modifier: ___________

15. A patient has a surgical procedure on Tuesday, and later that day the physician must take the patient back to the operating room to repeat (redo) a coronary bypass, due to complications of initial procedure.

    Modifier: ___________

16. The patient underwent a bilateral tympanoplasty.

    Modifier: ___________

17. If you must use two or more modifiers to describe a service, you would use which modifier to indicate this circumstance?

    Modifier: ___________

18. A surgeon performs a procedure on a neonate weighing 9 kg; the procedure was extremely complicated. What modifier would you use to indicate this service, which has an increased level of complexity?

    Modifier: ___________

19. Dr. Storely performed cataract surgery on 10/31/20XX, and Dr. Jones provided postoperative care following discharge. What modifier would you use to indicate the postoperative care following discharge?

    Modifier: ___________

Odd-numbered answers are located in Appendix B.

20. Dr. Merideth serves as an assistant surgeon to Dr. Taylor. What modifier would you add to the procedure code to indicate Dr. Merideth's status during the procedure?

    Modifier: ___________

21. The third-party payer requires the use of HCPCS/National modifiers; the surgeon performed a surgical procedure on the patient's left thumb. What Level II modifier would indicate the left thumb?

    Modifier: ___________

22. What Level II modifier indicates the upper left eyelid?

    Modifier: ___________

Odd-numbered answers are located in Appendix B.

CHAPTER 11

Evaluation and Management (E/M) Services

http://evolve.elsevier.com/Buck/step

THEORY

Without the use of reference material, complete the following:

1. _____ Consultation
2. _____ Admission
3. _____ Office visit
4. _____ Newborn care
5. _____ Established patient
6. _____ Inpatient
7. _____ New patient
8. _____ Outpatient

a. A face-to-face encounter in an office between the physician and patient

b. One who has not received professional service from the physician or another physician in the exact same specialty and subspecialty in the same group within the last 3 years

c. Advice or opinion from one physician to another physician

d. One who has been formally admitted to an acute health care facility

e. One who has received professional service from the physician or another physician in the exact same specialty and subspecialty in the same group within the last 3 years

f. Attention to an acute illness or injury that results in hospitalization

g. Evaluation and determination of care for a newborn infant

h. One who has not been formally admitted to a health care facility

Odd-numbered answers are located in Appendix B.

The four types of medical decision making, in order of complexity from most to least complex, are as follows:

9. ______________________________

10. ______________________________

11. ______________________________

12. ______________________________

13. Complexity of medical decision making is based on three

______________________________.

List the five types of presenting problems from the most risk and least recovery to least risk and most recovery:

14. ______________________________

15. ______________________________

16. ______________________________

17. ______________________________

18. ______________________________

19. Time that is used as a guide for outpatient services is what kind of time?

____

Provider time spent ordering medication and tests during or after

the visit is what kind of time? ______________________________

20. The patient's ______________ ______________ will reflect the number of systems examined by a brief statement of the findings.

21. A discussion with a patient and/or family concerning one or more of the following areas: diagnostic results, impressions and/or recommended diagnostic studies; prognosis; risks and benefits of treatment; instructions for treatment; importance of compliance with treatment; risk factor reduction; and patient and family education is

______________________________.

22. The history is the ______________ information the patient tells the physician.

Odd-numbered answers are located in Appendix B.

23. There is no distinction made between the new and established patients in this service department of a hospital: ____________________

24. Those services rendered by a physician whose opinion or advice is requested by another physician or agency in the evaluation and/or treatment of a patient is a(n) ______________, whereas the physician who has primary responsibility for the patient in the hospital is called ______________.

25. When critically ill patients in medical emergencies require the constant attendance of the physician (e.g., cardiac arrest, shock, bleeding, and respiratory failure) to stabilize them, what kind of care is needed?

____

26. When care is provided for similar services (e.g., hospital visits) to the same patient by more than one physician on the same day for different conditions, the care is ______________________________.

27. What is the name for the assumption of the total or specific care of a patient from one physician to another that does not constitute a consultation? ______________________________

28. If the physician who is standing by does so for 25 minutes, can he or she round the time up to 30 minutes for reporting purposes?

____

PRACTICAL

Office or Other Outpatient Services and Hospital Inpatient Service

With the use of the CPT and ICD-10-CM manuals, complete the following:

29. Analyze this case in which the patient record states: 40-year-old male patient (new) is evaluated for contusion of a finger. The history and examination are performed.

    a. Diagnosis and management options for contusion of finger. (Options can be minimal, limited, multiple, or extensive.) Diagnosis and management options: ______________

Odd-numbered answers are located in Appendix B.

Data to review to provide service. (Data can be minimal/none, limited, moderate, or extensive.) Only data available are current information obtained during the visit. Data: ________________

b. Risks if left untreated. (Risk can be minimal, low, moderate, or high.)

Risks: ________________

c. All three of the elements have been met to qualify this patient for what level of decision making complexity? ____________________

____

d. The patient record indicates that a history and examination were done. Considering the level of decision making complexity you arrived at for this patient, what is the correct CPT code for the case?

Code: ________________

30. A patient who was on observation status is discharged from the hospital. The patient was being observed after an automobile accident for subdural hematoma, subsequently ruled out. Code only the discharge services and diagnosis.

CPT Code: ________________

ICD-10-CM Codes: ______________, ______________

31. Initial observation of a patient was for upper abdominal pain, dizziness, and anemia. Moderate complexity decision making was conducted to admit the patient to observation to treat and rule out causes of the patient's anemia.

CPT Code: ________________

32. A 16-year-old female is being admitted by her family practice physician with a 2-week history of fatigue and fever. It has been progressively getting worse. She is suffering from dehydration. The physician performs a comprehensive history to look for explanations for her fatigue, including recent activity level and recent sleep habits. A detailed examination is performed, and she is diagnosed with mononucleosis and admitted for treatment.

CPT Code: ________________

ICD-10-CM Codes: ______________, ______________

Odd-numbered answers are located in Appendix B.

33. A 56-year-old male with an established history of ASHD of native arteries and past stent placement is admitted through the emergency room with acute onset of chest pain. An ECG was performed and troponin levels taken. Both showed evidence of the patient having an acute transmural inferior wall myocardial infarction with ST elevation. The cardiologist performs a comprehensive history, with the chief complaint, for the history of present illness (HPI), a complete review of systems (ROS), and past, family, and social history (PFSH). The history includes the information that the pain started a week ago but last night worsened. Also on a scale of 1 to 10, he rated the pain an 8. It was also discovered that the patient has not been attending regular appointments in the clinic setting. A comprehensive examination was performed along with high-complexity medical decision making (MDM), including management of the patient's acute MI and reviewing data of the medical history of the patient. He was taken immediately to the cardiac catheterization lab to look for the source for the patient's MI.

    CPT Code: ______________

    ICD-10-CM Codes: ______________, ______________, ______________

34. The patient is a 34-year-old established patient seen in the clinic by her dermatologist. She is followed for extensive plaque psoriasis involving her scalp, trunk, and arms. It has now worsened and spread to her palms, and she is now also complaining of joint pain. The spread to her hands has made it difficult to do many of her day-to-day tasks. A history and examination are performed. The examination includes inspection of the affected areas in addition to bending and rotation of joints. A long discussion took place regarding a change in her medications to try to gain better control of her psoriasis and slow down the systemic progression. Topical and systemic treatment was decided on. Total time spent was 35 minutes.

    CPT Code: ________________

    ICD-10-CM Codes: ______________, ______________

35. A 2-year-old boy with bacterial pneumonia is hospitalized and has had 5 days of antibiotic therapy. Today the child developed a fever of 101° F with a mild rash on his torso. In a subsequent hospital visit, the attending physician performed a problem-focused history and examination. The MDM complexity was low.

    CPT Code: ______________

    ICD-10-CM Code: ______________

Odd-numbered answers are located in Appendix B.

36. The patient is a 52-year-old male from out of state visiting his daughter. He left his medications for his benign hypertension at home and is now here in the clinic in need of a prescription. A history and examination are performed, and straightforward MDM. A prescription is given to the patient.

    CPT Code: ___________________

    ICD-10-CM Code: ________________

Consultation Services

37. A 47-year-old female was sent by her family practice physician for an office consultation with a gynecologist. The patient has been suffering with moderate pelvic pain, a heavy sensation in her lower pelvis, and marked discomfort during sexual intercourse. In a detailed history, the gynecologist noted the location, severity, and duration of her pelvic pain and related symptoms. In the review of systems, the patient had positive findings related to her gastrointestinal, genitourinary, and endocrine body systems. The physician noted that her medical history was noncontributory to the present problem. The detailed physical examination centered on her gastrointestinal and genitourinary systems, with a complete pelvic examination. The physician ordered laboratory tests and a pelvic ultrasound to determine uterine fibroids, endometritis, or other internal gynecological pathology. The MDM complexity was moderate.

    CPT Code: ___________________

    ICD-10-CM Codes: ________________, ________________

38. A 38-year-old female has severe low back pain due to a trauma injury she experienced as a factory worker 4 years ago. The chronic pain has become almost unbearable, and her internal medicine physician cannot go any further with her treatment. An initial outpatient consultation is requested, and the patient is sent to see the pain management specialist for suggestions to control the chronic pain. A comprehensive history is taken, including all of the pertinent information regarding her injury. During the comprehensive examination the patient's gait and movement were observed. Moderate-complexity decision making is performed, including different treatment options. A separate note is dictated to show the requesting physician what results were found during the visit and the decision on treatment of her pain.

    CPT Code: ___________________

    ICD-10-CM Codes: ________________, ________________

39. An inpatient urological consultation is performed for a 32-year-old female who recently had an elective abortion performed on an outpatient basis. The woman has been admitted with a high fever, pelvic pain, and dysuria. During a detailed history, the urologist notes in the

Odd-numbered answers are located in Appendix B.

history of present illness that the patient's symptoms began about 2 days after the abortion and progressed to the acute phase, which she is in at the present time. The location of the pain is in the lower abdomen and rated 9 on a scale of 1 to 10. She reports the quality of the pain to be sharp and stabbing. In the review of systems, the physician notes positive responses in 5 of the 12 body systems investigated. The urologist notes a negative medical history related to urinary symptoms other than a mild cystitis about 10 years ago. The detailed physical examination performed by the urologist centers on the genitourinary system and gastrointestinal system in significant detail. The medical decision making is low. Given the patient's past surgical procedure and physical findings at the present, the consultant considers the diagnoses of pyelonephritis, cystitis, pyelitis, and endometritis.

CPT Code: ___________________

40. A 46-year-old male is admitted to the hospital with a progressive staphylococcal pneumonia that is not responding to treatment. A request is made for the infectious disease physician on staff to render his opinion for treatment. The patient is seen in initial inpatient consultation. An expanded problem-focused history and examination are performed. After looking at the sputum cultures, the physician decides on the most effective antibiotic for treatment. The decision making is straightforward.

CPT Code: ___________________

ICD-10-CM Code: ________________

41. The initial consulting physician subsequently sees a 55-year-old patient injured at work when he fell from a house roof and struck his head. The patient had a right frontal parietal craniotomy 6 days previously and is recovering rapidly. The initial consultation was requested regarding a possible drug reaction that produced a rash on the upper torso. The consultant recommended a medication change, but after 48 hours the patient had no improvement. The physician re-evaluates for other possible causes of the rash. An expanded problem-focused interval history and a physical examination were performed. The MDM complexity was moderate.

CPT Code: ___________________

ICD-10-CM Code: ________________

42. A 44-year-old patient, with chronic mastoiditis, was seen in consultation by the ENT specialist in the office. Her physician was inquiring as to the advantages of surgery versus continued antibiotic treatment when an acute flare comes on. The ENT specialist recommends surgery because of the increasing severity with each acute flare. She is fearful of the surgery because of the need to go under

Odd-numbered answers are located in Appendix B.

general anesthetic and a fear of permanent hearing loss. The physician performs an expanded problem-focused history to include the duration of this problem and how many acute flares a year the patient experiences. An expanded problem-focused examination and straightforward decision making are completed. It is determined that with the number of acute flares a year and the increasing severity of each case that surgery is recommended. The patient's fears are laid to rest, and the patient decides to go ahead with the surgery.

CPT Code: ___________________

ICD-10-CM Code: _______________

43. This is a follow-up visit on a 28-year-old male who is admitted with the diagnosis of headaches. The patient is subsequently seen because the physician needs to follow up on test results that weren't back yet at the initial consultation. This will help to find a possible cause of the headaches and course of treatment. A problem-focused history and examination and low-complexity decision making are made after viewing the CT results. The diagnosis of tension headaches was made and treatment options discussed.

CPT Code: ___________________

ICD-10-CM Code: _______________

44. An 83-year-old patient is seen at the local nursing home. The patient suffers from severe COPD. Routine labs were drawn on the patient by her primary doctor, and her blood sugar came back abnormal. Fasting glucose was then taken and was high. The endocrinologist was asked to render an opinion on a possible diagnosis of diabetes. A problem-focused history and examination and straightforward decision making were made. Diabetes was diagnosed and treatment started. The endocrinologist contacted the primary physician and discussed treatment of the patient. Report services for the endocrinologist only.

CPT Code: ___________________

ICD-10-CM Code: _______________

45. A patient is sent to a general surgeon by her family physician for an opinion and recommendation for surgical repair of a recurrent femoral hernia, right. A brief problem-focused history of present illness and a problem-focused examination of the affected body area and organ system are performed in the office. The MDM complexity was straightforward.

CPT Code: ___________________

ICD-10-CM Code: _______________

Odd-numbered answers are located in Appendix B.

46. A pulmonologist is asked by the patient's primary physician to see a 14-month-old boy who was admitted to the hospital with respiratory distress, cough, and fever. A comprehensive history is taken from the parents because this is an infant. It was determined that the patient does attend a day care facility. The cough and fever have been present for approximately 5 days. The infant started having trouble breathing this morning. The patient is intubated. Pneumonia due to respiratory syncytial virus is the definitive diagnosis. A comprehensive examination is performed along with moderate decision making. More tests will follow. A copy of his dictation will be sent to the primary physician.

    CPT Code: ____________________

    ICD-10-CM Code: ________________

47. Office neurosurgery consultation is requested by the primary physician for a 32-year-old man on workers' compensation who is unable to work because of displacement of intervertebral lumbar disc with myelopathy. Two previous surgical repairs have been unsuccessful in relieving the patient's pain. The patient has been unable to return to his employment as a bricklayer. He complains of radiating pain throughout the buttocks and leg, with numbness throughout the leg and foot. Reflexes are minimal to nonexistent. A comprehensive history and physical examination are performed. MDM complexity was high due to the prior surgeries and continued complaints.

    CPT Code: ____________________

    ICD-10-CM Code: ________________

Emergency Department Services, Nursing Facility, Domiciliary, and Home Services

48. A patient presents to the emergency department after being involved in a motor vehicle accident. The patient was wearing a seat belt. The vehicle rolled numerous times. The patient's head struck the side window. The patient is unresponsive and is intubated. A history was unable to be obtained because of the patient's unresponsiveness. What history is available comes from the paramedics and patient's record. A comprehensive examination reveals the abdomen to be quite swollen with extensive bruising around the lower abdomen caused by the seat belt. High-complexity decision making was involved, and the patient was rushed to the operating room.

    CPT Code: ____________________

Odd-numbered answers are located in Appendix B.

49. A male patient presents to the emergency department with a wrist sprain sustained in a softball game when the patient slid into home, striking his hand on home plate. The patient is in apparent pain with a swollen wrist, which he is unable to flex. A history and physical examination are done. Radiographs show a Colles' fracture of the distal radius. The MDM complexity was low.

CPT Code: ________________

ICD-10-CM Codes: ______________, ______________, ______________

50. An 88-year-old female's family physician comes to the nursing facility to perform the resident's annual exam. A detailed interval history is taken with some information from the patient, but because of her limited cognitive abilities, most of the information is gathered from the nurses and past records. A comprehensive multisystem physical examination is performed, which includes extensive body areas and related organ systems. The MDM complexity was moderate because multiple diagnoses must be considered for this patient, who has senile dementia, diabetes, hypertension, hypothyroidism, and recurrent transient ischemic attacks. The creation of a new treatment plan is required because some of the patient's conditions have worsened.

CPT Code: ________________

ICD-10-CM Codes: ______________, ______________,

______________, ________________, ________________

51. This is a home visit on an elderly gentleman, previously unknown to me, who is complaining of edema in his lower extremities. Pain is associated with this. Low-complexity decision making for this visit. Jobst stockings are prescribed.

CPT Code: ________________

ICD-10-CM Code: ______________

52. Subsequent follow-up care is provided for the 82-year-old male nursing facility patient with Alzheimer's disease. The resident has responded well to some new medications and appears to have recovered some of his cognitive abilities without behavioral disturbances. The physician performs a problem-focused history and physical examination on his neurological problem and orders the current treatments continued. The MDM complexity is low.

CPT Code: ________________

ICD-10-CM Codes: ______________, ______________

Odd-numbered answers are located in Appendix B.

53. Subsequent follow-up care is provided for the patient who was transferred to a skilled nursing facility from an acute care hospital after partial recovery from a stroke. The patient has developed periods of extreme dizziness and mental confusion. A detailed interval history is gathered, and a detailed physical examination of the affected body systems is performed. Given the possibility that a new stroke could have occurred or that other neurological problems have developed, new orders are written, and the physician plans to return the next day to evaluate the patient's condition again. The MDM complexity is moderate.

    CPT Code: ________________

    ICD-10-CM Codes: ______________, ______________, ______________

54. The physician provides services to a resident of a rest home for an ulcerative sore on the heel and midfoot. Given the fact that the patient is in reasonably good health and is not diabetic, the physician focuses his attention on the right lower extremity during the problem-focused physical examination. The physician knows the resident well and performs a brief HPI and ROS during a problem-focused history. The resident thinks the sore is from new shoes, and the physician agrees with that conclusion. Topical antibiotic cream is ordered, and the new shoes are sent to the cobbler to be stretched. The MDM complexity is straightforward.

    CPT Code: ________________

    ICD-10-CM Code: ______________

55. The physician provides services to a new patient who is in a nursing facility. The patient is 43 years old and is paraplegic, with severe infected stasis ulcers. The physician performs a detailed history and examination and prescribes an antibiotic. The MDM was straightforward.

    CPT Code: ________________

Prolonged Services and Preventive Medicine Services

56. An established patient is seen in the office for a new problem that requires a history and examination. The MDM complexity is high, and the physician spends 40 minutes with the patient. However, the patient has numerous concerns, and the physician spends an additional hour and 50 minutes in prolonged direct patient contact.

    CPT Codes: ________________, ________________

Odd-numbered answers are located in Appendix B.

57. A 44-year-old asthmatic patient (new) is scheduled for a routine office visit for a complaint of severe headaches. The physician provides a history and examination. The MDM complexity was high. Toward the end of the visit, the patient develops severe breathing complications, and the physician spends the next hour and 30 minutes administering treatment.

    CPT Codes: ________________, ________________

58. A 64-year-old man arrives at his appointment with his family physician for his annual physical examination. The patient has no new complaints, and all of his medications remain the same. He is told to follow up in 1 year or sooner if necessary.

    CPT Code: ________________

Services from Throughout the E/M Section

59. A new patient is seen in the office for a variety of medical problems. The patient has insulin-dependent diabetes mellitus with complicating eye and renal problems. She also has hypertensive heart disease with episodes of congestive heart failure. Her peripheral vascular disease has worsened, and she can walk only a block before she is crippled with extreme leg pain. The patient reports that a new problem has surfaced: throbbing headaches with radiating neck pain. To manage and investigate the multiplicity of problems, the physician performs a history and physical examination. A complete review of systems is performed, as is an update to her complete past, family, and social history. The physician has to take a multitude of factors into consideration because this patient's problems are highly complex. Total time spent with the patient was 60 minutes.

    CPT Code: ________________

60. A new patient is seen in the office complaining of a sore throat and reports a low-grade fever for the past 4 days. The physician performs a history and an examination of the respiratory and lymphatic systems. The physician's impression was acute pharyngitis, and straightforward decision making was performed. Amoxicillin was prescribed.

    CPT Code: ________________

    ICD-10-CM Code: ______________

61. This is a 32-year-old female patient admitted for observation after an allergic reaction to her pain medication. She is alert and oriented, but has severe pruritus and shortness of breath. A detailed history and examination are performed after she takes medication for the pruritus;

Odd-numbered answers are located in Appendix B.

the breathing improved and the patient was discharged from observation on the same day.

CPT Code: ________________

ICD-10-CM Codes: ______________, ______________,

____

62. The patient was admitted to the hospital 3 days ago with severe dehydration and hyponatremia. The patient is now being discharged. Discharge takes 30 minutes.

CPT Code: ________________

ICD-10-CM Codes: ______________, ______________

63. A family practice physician who is treating a 20-year-old man (inpatient) for bronchitis calls in a urologist to examine the patient, who has requested a circumcision. The consultant performs a problem-focused history and problem-focused physical examination and determines that there is no urgency for the surgical procedure. The physician's decision making is fairly straightforward, and he recommends that the patient have the procedure done as an outpatient at a later date.

CPT Code: ________________

64. A physician visits a 75-year-old female in the extended nursing facility as part of her annual exam. The physician completes a detailed interval history with a comprehensive, head-to-toe physical examination. The physician reviews and affirms the medical plan of care developed by the multidisciplinary care team at the nursing facility. The patient's condition is stable; her hypertension and diabetes (type 2) are in good control, and she has no new problems. The physician has limited data to review and few diagnoses to consider. The MDM complexity was moderate.

CPT Code: ________________

ICD-10-CM Codes: ______________, ______________

65. A 67-year-old female is admitted with severe exacerbation of her COPD. The patient is now in respiratory failure and CHF. The patient is intubated and unconscious; 155 minutes of critical care time was spent at bedside and coordinating care for this patient.

CPT Code(s): ________________

ICD-10-CM Code(s): ______________

User to decide number of codes necessary to correctly answer the question.

Odd-numbered answers are located in Appendix B.

66. Henry Green, an established patient, came into the office for his yearly physical examination. Henry is 72 and in good health.

    CPT Code: ____________________

    ICD-10-CM Code: ________________

REPORTS

In Appendix A of this workbook you will find a section titled Reports, which contains original reports. Read the reports indicated below and supply the appropriate CPT and ICD-10-CM codes on the following lines:

67. Report 1

    CPT Code: ____________________

    ICD-10-CM Codes: ________________, ________________,

    ____

68. Report 2

    CPT Code: ____________________

    ICD-10-CM Codes: ________________(secondary neoplasm),

    ________________ (primary neoplasm), ________________ (vena

    cava syndrome), ________________ (catheter complication),

    ________________ (hypertension), ________________ (nerve pain),

    ________________ (anemia, in (due to) (with), neoplastic disease)

69. Report 3

    CPT Code: ____________________

    ICD-10-CM Code: ________________

70. Report 4

    CPT Code: ____________________

71. Report 5

    CPT Code: ____________________

Odd-numbered answers are located in Appendix B.

Anesthesia

http://evolve.elsevier.com/Buck/step

THEORY

Without the use of reference material, answer the following:

1. What two words describe a decreased level of consciousness that does not put patients completely to sleep and that allows the patients to breathe on their own during a surgical procedure? ________________ ________________
2. What do the initials CRNA stand for?

    ____
3. CMS publishes an annual list of ________________ values for anesthesia codes.
4. The "M" in the anesthesia formula stands for ________________ unit.
5. What is the term that describes the services provided to a patient by the physician before surgery?

    ____
6. What is the term for the time after surgery when the physician provides services to the patient?

    ____
7. The ________________ factor for the locale is multiplied by the number of base units in the procedure plus the time units to determine the price of the anesthesia service.
8. This modifier indicates that a CRNA service with medical direction by a physician was provided. __________

Odd-numbered answers are located in Appendix B.

PRACTICAL

With the use of the CPT manual, identify the following physical status modifiers:

9. Patient with a severe systemic disease that is a constant threat to life.

   Modifier: ___________

10. Normal healthy patient.

    Modifier: ___________

11. Patient with a severe systemic disease.

    Modifier: ___________

12. Declared brain-dead patient whose organs are being removed for donor purposes.

    Modifier: ___________

13. Patient with mild systemic disease.

    Modifier: ___________

14. Moribund patient who is not expected to survive without the operation.

    Modifier: ___________

Locate anesthesia procedures in the CPT manual index under the entry "Anesthesia" and then subtermed by the anatomic site. Write the CPT index location on the line provided (e.g., Anesthesia, Thyroid). Then locate the code identified in the anesthesia section of the CPT manual. Choose the correct code, and write the code on the line provided.

15. Diagnostic arthroscopic procedure of knee joint.

    Index location: _________________

    CPT Code: _________________

16. Radical hysterectomy.

    Index location: _________________

    CPT Code: _________________

17. Corneal transplant.

    Index location: _________________

    CPT Code: _________________

Odd-numbered answers are located in Appendix B.

18. Cesarean delivery only.

    Index location: ________________

    CPT Code: ________________

19. Otoscopy used in procedure for middle ear.

    Index location: ________________

    CPT Code: ________________

20. Transurethral resection of the prostate.

    Index location: ________________

    CPT Code: ________________

21. Anesthesia for a cardiac catheterization patient having mild systemic disease.

    CPT Code: ________________

22. Anesthesia for a myringotomy on a healthy 5-year-old patient.

    CPT Code: ________________

Assign the diagnosis code(s) for Questions 23–26.

23. Diverticulitis of colon with hemorrhage.

    ICD-10-CM Code: ______________

24. Atherosclerosis of coronary artery bypass graft utilizing internal mammary artery.

    ICD-10-CM Code: ______________

25. Toxic diffuse goiter with thyrotoxic crisis.

    ICD-10-CM Code: ______________

26. Mitral valve regurgitation as a late effect of Fen-Phen, taken as prescribed, initial encounter.

    ICD-10-CM Codes: ______________, ______________

Odd-numbered answers are located in Appendix B.

REPORTS

In Appendix A of this workbook you will find a section titled Reports, which contains original reports. Read the reports indicated below and supply the appropriate CPT anesthesia codes on the following lines:

27. Report 7

    CPT Code: ____________________

28. Report 41

    CPT Code: ____________________

29. Report 44

    CPT Codes: ____________________, ____________________

30. Report 83

    CPT Code: ____________________

Odd-numbered answers are located in Appendix B.

CHAPTER 13

Surgery Guidelines and General Surgery

http://evolve.elsevier.com/Buck/step

THEORY

Without the use of reference material, answer the following:

1. The more complex subsections referred to in the text are Integumentary, Musculoskeletal, Respiratory, Cardiovascular, Digestive,

   and ____.

2. The information in the ______________ contains information that is necessary to correctly code in the section, and the information is not repeated elsewhere.

3. Notes may appear before subsections, subheadings, ______________, and subcategories within the CPT manual.

4. When a note is present, that note must be read and

   ______________ if the coding is to be accurate.

5. Within the Surgery Guidelines, the ______________ procedure codes are presented in a list by anatomic site.

6. According to the CPT manual, "Pertinent information [in the

   ______________ report] should include an adequate definition or description of the nature, extent, need, time, effort, and equipment necessary to provide the service."

7. There are minor and ______________ procedure designations for the purposes of a surgical package.

8. If a breast biopsy and mastectomy of the left breast were performed during the same operative session, would both procedures be reported?

   ____

9. If a breast biopsy and right knee operation were performed during the same operative session, would both procedures be reported?

   ____

Odd-numbered answers are located in Appendix B.

10. The CPT manual describes the surgical package as including one related preoperative E/M service, the operative procedure, and immediate

    ________________ care.

11. Local infiltration is considered ________________ anesthesia.

12. This term means a worsening as described in the text.

    ____

13. This type of anesthesia is not part of the surgical package.

    ____

14. The predefined number of days before and after a surgical procedure are referred to as the ________________ period.

15. What is the CPT code that reports a surgical tray? ________________

16. What is the HCPCS code that reports a surgical tray?

    ____

17. According to the Medicare guidelines, a surgical package includes the treatment of complications by the ________________ physician.

18. At an office visit, a decision for surgery was made. The surgical procedure was scheduled 21 days later. Would the office visit service be:
    a. Reported separately
    b. Included in the surgical procedure

19. Splitting open of the surgical wound is ________________.

20. Inclusion or exclusion of a procedure in the CPT manual implies health insurance coverage or no health insurance coverage.

    True or False? __________

PRACTICAL

With the use of a CPT manual, answer the following:

21. The code range in the Surgical section is ________________ to ________________.

22. The subsection that follows the Digestive System is the ________________ System.

Odd-numbered answers are located in Appendix B.

23. What type of microscope has a subsection of the Surgery section?

____

24. The difference between 10005 and 10021 is that one is with

____________________ ____________________ and one is without it.

25. According to the parenthetical information following code 10012, for a percutaneous needle biopsy other than fine needle aspiration, see

____________________ for salivary gland.

26. According to the Surgery Guidelines, codes designated as

"____________________ ____________________" should not be reported in addition to the code for the total procedure or service of which it is considered an integral component.

27. According to the Surgery Guidelines, follow-up care for

____________________ surgical procedures includes only that care which is usually a part of the surgical procedure.

28. According to the Surgery Guidelines, the code range for Maternity Care

and Delivery is ____________________-____________________.

29. According to the Surgery Guidelines, this is the code for unlisted

procedures of the lip. ____________________

30. According to the Surgery Guidelines, this is the code for unlisted

procedures of the urinary system. ____________________

Odd-numbered answers are located in Appendix B.

CHAPTER 14

Integumentary System

http://evolve.elsevier.com/Buck/step

THEORY

Integumentary System Terminology

Match the following terms to the correct definitions:

1. _____ Dermis
2. _____ Epidermis
3. _____ Subcutaneous
4. _____ Incision and drainage
5. _____ Abscess
6. _____ Cyst
7. _____ Debridement
8. _____ Paring
9. _____ Biopsy
10. _____ Shaving

a. Localized collection of pus that will result in the disintegration of tissue over time

b. Second layer of skin holding blood vessels, nerve endings, sweat glands, and hair follicles

c. Removal of a small piece of living tissue for diagnostic purposes

d. Outer layer of skin

e. Horizontal or transverse removal of dermal or epidermal lesions, without full-thickness excision

f. Cleansing of or removing dead tissue from a wound

g. To cut and withdraw fluid

h. Removal of thin layers of skin by peeling or scraping

i. Tissue below dermis, primarily fat cells that insulate the body

j. Closed sac containing matter or fluid

Odd-numbered answers are located in Appendix B.

Match the following terms to the correct definitions:

11. _____ Excision
12. _____ Benign
13. _____ Malignant
14. _____ Repair
15. _____ Skin graft
16. _____ Tissue transfer
17. _____ Destruction
18. _____ Mast-
19. _____ Cryosurgery

a. Full-thickness removal of a lesion that may include simple closure
b. Prefix meaning breast
c. Transplantation of tissue to repair a defect
d. Not progressive or recurrent
e. Killing of tissue, possibly by electrocautery, laser, chemical, or other means
f. Destruction of lesions using extreme cold
g. Pertains to suturing a wound
h. Piece of skin for grafting that is still partially attached to the original blood supply and is used to cover an adjacent wound area
i. Used to describe a cancerous tumor that grows worse over time

20. If multiple lesions are treated, the most complex lesion is listed first and the others are usually listed using modifier:
    a. -50
    b. -51
    c. -47
    d. -99

21. This condition is chronic abscessing and subsequent infection of a sweat gland.
    a. Folliculitis
    b. Hyperhidrosis
    c. Miliaria
    d. Hidradenitis

22. An example of a corn or callus is a benign:
    a. Hyperkeratotic skin lesion
    b. Lipoma or dermatofibroma
    c. Nevi or dysplastic nevi
    d. Dermoid cyst or nevi or dysplastic nevi

Odd-numbered answers are located in Appendix B.

PRACTICAL

Using the CPT and ICD-10-CM manuals, code the following services:

23. Joan, an established patient, comes into the office to have an intermediate repair of a 2.6 cm wound on her right arm. A surgical tray was used.

    CPT Codes: ________________, ________________

    ICD-10-CM Code: ______________

24. Rita, an established patient, has a 16.2 cm simple repair of the cheek. A surgical tray is used.

    CPT Codes: ________________, ________________

    ICD-10-CM Code: ______________

25. Lisa, an established patient, has a percutaneous biopsy with stereotactic image guidance for a left breast mass. A surgical tray was used. The pathology report later indicated a neoplasm of uncertain behavior.

    CPT Codes: ________________, ________________

    ICD-10-CM Code: ______________

26. What code would be used to report Mr. Jones's visit to Dr. Green 2 weeks after major surgery?

    CPT Code: ________________

    ICD-10-CM Code: ______________

27. Excision axillary hidradenitis, complex repair.

    CPT Code: ________________

    ICD-10-CM Code: ______________

28. Debridement; 16 sq cm subcutaneous tissue and muscle due to a diabetic foot ulcer.

    CPT Code: ________________

    ICD-10-CM Codes: ______________, ______________

29. Removal of tissue expander without insertion of prosthesis.

    CPT Code: ________________

30. Excision of abscessed pilonidal cyst; complicated.

    CPT Code: ________________

    ICD-10-CM Code: ______________

Odd-numbered answers are located in Appendix B.

31. Removal of subdermal contraceptive implant.

    CPT Code: ________________

    ICD-10-CM Code: ______________

32. Debridement of four fingernails due to onychomycosis.

    CPT Code: ________________

    ICD-10-CM Code: ______________

33. Excision of 4 cm benign lesion of face (most resource intensive) and excision of 3 cm benign lesion of neck.

    CPT Code(s): ________________

    ICD-10-CM Code(s): ______________

34. Excision of a 2.5 cm malignant lip lesion and two malignant lesions of the skin of the chest, each 1.5 cm in diameter.

    CPT Code(s): ________________

    ICD-10-CM Code(s): ______________

35. Destruction by laser of three premalignant actinic keratosis facial lesions.

    CPT Code(s): ________________

    ICD-10-CM Code(s): ______________

36. Destruction of 4.0 cm malignant lesion of the eyelid.

    CPT Code(s): ________________

    ICD-10-CM Code(s): ______________

37. Suzanne Osterland, a 4-year-old, is brought to the office by her father. Suzanne was playing on the swing set at the playground when she fell approximately 5 feet from the top step of the play set. When she fell, she struck her leg on a birdbath rim and then on the playground gardener's pail with several garden forks protruding over the rim, sustaining 12.9 cm, 3.1 cm, and 2.1 cm lacerations of the lower right leg, requiring deep-layers of subcutaneous closure and non-muscle fascia accomplished after subcutaneous tissue debridement of 18 sq cm.

    CPT Codes: ________________, ________________

    ICD-10-CM Codes: ________________, ______________ (W code),

    ______________ (W code), ______________ (Y code)

User to decide number of codes necessary to correctly answer the question.

Odd-numbered answers are located in Appendix B.

38. Electrosurgical destruction of a 1.0 cm malignant lesion of the neck.

CPT Code(s): ____________________

ICD-10-CM Code(s): ________________

39. Cryosurgical destruction of 10 flat warts on the hand.

CPT Code(s): ____________________

ICD-10-CM Code(s): ________________

40. Laser destruction of multiple malignant lesions, as follows: 3.4 cm on right hand, 2.1 cm on left hand, 5.2 cm on right hand, 4.3 cm on left hand, 0.3 cm on right upper eyelid, 0.5 cm on left upper eyelid.

CPT Code(s): ____________________

ICD-10-CM Code(s): ________________

41. Debridement of back for extensive eczematous skin, 20% body surface.

CPT Code(s): ____________________

ICD-10-CM Code(s): ________________

42. Bilateral blepharoplasty of upper eyelid due to ptosis.

CPT Code(s): ____________________

ICD-10-CM Code(s): ________________

43. Initial, local treatment, first-degree burn, of back of hand, 5% body surface. The burn was caused by steam from a pipe at his home that accidentally was connected improperly.

CPT Code(s): ____________________

ICD-10-CM Code(s): ________________

44. Mohs micrographic surgery of arm for a poorly defined malignant neoplasm, first stage, 4 tissue blocks.

CPT Code(s): ____________________

ICD-10-CM Code(s): ________________

45. Mastotomy with drainage of deep abscess.

CPT Code(s): ____________________

ICD-10-CM Code(s): ________________

User to decide number of codes necessary to correctly answer the question.

Odd-numbered answers are located in Appendix B.

REPORTS

In Appendix A of this workbook you will find a section titled Reports, which contains original reports. Read the reports indicated below and supply the appropriate CPT and ICD-10-CM codes on the following lines:

46. Report 6

    CPT Code(s): ____________________

    ICD-10-CM Code(s): ________________

47. Report 7

    CPT Code(s): ____________________

    ICD-10-CM Code(s): ________________

48. Report 8

    CPT Code(s): ____________________

    ICD-10-CM Code(s): ________________

49. Report 9

    CPT Code(s): ____________________

    ICD-10-CM Code(s): ________________

50. Report 11

    CPT Code(s): ____________________

    ICD-10-CM Code(s): ________________

51. Report 12

    CPT Code(s): ____________________

    ICD-10-CM Code(s): ________________

User to decide number of codes necessary to correctly answer the question.

Odd-numbered answers are located in Appendix B.

Musculoskeletal System

http://evolve.elsevier.com/Buck/step

THEORY

Musculoskeletal Terminology

Without the use of reference material, match the following terms to the correct definitions:

1. _____ Closed treatment
2. _____ Open treatment
3. _____ Percutaneous
4. _____ Fracture
5. _____ Dislocation
6. _____ Manipulation
7. _____ Fixation
8. _____ Skeletal traction
9. _____ Soft tissue
10. _____ Arthroplasty
11. _____ Arthrodesis

a. Application of force to a limb with the use of a pin, screw, wire, or clamp attached to the bone
b. Displacement of a bone from its normal location in a joint
c. The application of pins, wires, screws, and so on to immobilize; these can be placed externally or internally
d. Fracture treatment when site is not surgically opened and visualized or reduced
e. Word used interchangeably with reduction to mean the attempted restoration of a fracture or joint dislocation to its normal anatomic position
f. Fracture site that is surgically opened and visualized
g. Surgical immobilization of a joint
h. Tissues (fascia, connective tissue, muscle, etc.) surrounding organs and other structures
i. Break in a bone
j. Fixation considered neither open nor closed; fracture is not visualized, but fixation is placed across the fracture site under x-ray imaging
k. Reshaping or reconstructing a joint

Odd-numbered answers are located in Appendix B.

Without the use of reference material, answer the following:

12. Would a biopsy code usually include the administration of any necessary local anesthesia? Yes or No? ___________

13. What is arthrocentesis? ___________

14. What is a uniplane fixation device? ___________

____

15. What is the name of the graft that is taken from the upper thigh area where the fascia is the thickest? ___________

16. What type of stimulation often is used to promote healing of a slow-healing fracture? ___________

17. What is fast becoming the surgical method of choice for many musculoskeletal procedures today? ___________

18. What is the term that describes the use of tape applied to the body to provide support or limit motion? ___________

19. Do you bill for the removal of a cast that your physician applied? Yes or No? ___________ Why or why not? ___________

____

20. What two words describe when elastic wrap or tape is fastened to the skin or wrapped around a limb and weights are then attached to the wraps or tape? ___________

21. What is the primary difference between the excision codes found in the Musculoskeletal System subsection and the excision codes found in the Integumentary System subsection? ___________

____

____

Odd-numbered answers are located in Appendix B.

PRACTICAL

With the use of the CPT and ICD-10-CM manual(s), code the following:

22. John is returning to the physician's office 2 weeks postsurgery for an application of a new long-leg cast. The patient required surgery due to a traumatic fracture of the lower leg.

    CPT Code: ________________

    ICD-10-CM Codes: ______________, ______________

23. Julie Mason, age 5 years, is coming in today to have her long-arm cast removed and replaced with a short-arm cast for 3 weeks. The patient sustained a torus fracture of the upper end of the radius and is 1 week postop.

    CPT Code: ________________

    ICD-10-CM Codes: ______________, ______________

24. Jamie Larson slipped on the ice and twisted her knee when she fell. During diagnostic arthroscopy, a bucket-handle tear of the medial and lateral meniscus was seen and repaired.

    CPT Code: ________________

    ICD-10-CM Codes: ______________, ______________, ______________

25. Percutaneous skeletal fixation of closed calcaneal fracture requiring manipulation.

    CPT Code: ________________

    ICD-10-CM Code: ______________

26. Closed treatment of multiple pelvic fractures without displacement of the pelvic ring; without manipulation.

    CPT Code: ________________

    ICD-10-CM Code: ______________

27. Closed treatment of a single closed metacarpophalangeal dislocation, distal end; with manipulation and without anesthesia.

    CPT Code: ________________

    ICD-10-CM Code: ______________

Odd-numbered answers are located in Appendix B.

28. Open treatment of a closed traumatic anterior hip dislocation without fixation.

    CPT Code: ________________

    ICD-10-CM Code: ______________

29. Closed treatment of a patellar fracture; no manipulation.

    CPT Code: ________________

    ICD-10-CM Code: ______________

30. Closed treatment of a closed patellar dislocation; no anesthesia.

    CPT Code: ________________

    ICD-10-CM Code: ______________

31. Manipulation of a knee joint under general anesthesia with application of a traction device. Patient had an anterior dislocation of the tibia, proximal end.

    CPT Code: ________________

    ICD-10-CM Code: ______________

32. Closed treatment of a closed tarsal bone dislocation without anesthesia.

    CPT Code: ________________

    ICD-10-CM Code: ______________

33. Depressed frontal sinus fracture repaired using open treatment.

    CPT Code: ________________

34. Open treatment of a Le Fort I maxillary fracture.

    CPT Code: ________________

35. Aspiration and injection of a bone cyst.

    CPT Code: ________________

36. Removal of deep screws from a repaired fracture. (The screws are fixation devices.)

    CPT Code: ________________

Odd-numbered answers are located in Appendix B.

37. Replantation of index finger, including sublimis tendon insertion, following a complete traumatic amputation. Code only the replantation service.

    CPT Code: ________________

38. Costochondral cartilage graft.

    CPT Code: ________________

39. Therapeutic injection of corticosteroids for medial nerve entrapment (CTS).

    CPT Code: ________________

    ICD-10-CM Code: ______________

40. Aspiration of a shoulder joint.

    CPT Code: ________________

41. Removal of a halo that was applied by another physician.

    CPT Code: ________________

42. Subsequent removal of a short-arm cast by the physician who applied the cast.

    CPT Code: ________________

43. Closed treatment of a mandibular fracture without manipulation.

    CPT Code: ________________

44. Application of a shoulder-to-hip body cast.

    CPT Code: ________________

45. Wedging of a clubfoot cast.

    CPT Code: ________________

46. Application of a short-leg splint.

    CPT Code: ________________

47. Strapping of a hip.

    CPT Code: ________________

Odd-numbered answers are located in Appendix B.

48. Application of a long-arm splint.

    CPT Code: ________________

49. Strapping of a 40-year-old's thorax.

    CPT Code: ________________

50. Surgical arthroscopy of the temporomandibular joint.

    CPT Code: ________________

51. Application, cast; figure-of-eight.

    CPT Code: ________________

52. Surgical arthroscopy, elbow; limited debridement.

    CPT Code: ________________

53. Diagnostic hip arthroscopy.

    CPT Code: ________________

54. Surgical arthroscopy with lateral meniscus repair of knee.

    CPT Code: ________________

55. Arthroscopic chondroplasty of knee with minimal debridement.

    CPT Code: ________________

56. Endoscopic plantar fasciotomy.

    CPT Code: ________________

57. Release of a transverse carpal ligament of the wrist with surgical endoscopy.

    CPT Code: ________________

58. Arthrocentesis of ganglion cyst of toe joint, both injection and aspiration.

    CPT Code: ________________

    ICD-10-CM Code: ______________

59. Excision of maxillary torus palatinus.

    CPT Code: ____________________

Odd-numbered answers are located in Appendix B.

REPORTS

In Appendix A of this workbook you will find a section titled Reports, which contains original reports. Read the reports indicated below and supply the appropriate CPT and ICD-10-CM codes on the following lines:

60. Report 10

    CPT Code: __________________

    ICD-10-CM Codes: __________________, ________________,

    __________________ (External Cause code)

61. Report 13

    CPT Code: __________________

    ICD-10-CM Code: ______________

62. Report 14

    CPT Code: __________________

    ICD-10-CM Codes: ______________, ______________

63. Report 15

    CPT Code: __________________

    ICD-10-CM Codes: ______________, ______________

64. Report 16

    CPT Code: __________________

    ICD-10-CM Codes: ______________, ______________

65. Report 17

    CPT Code: __________________

    ICD-10-CM Code: ______________

66. Report 18

    CPT Code: __________________

    ICD-10-CM Code: ______________

Odd-numbered answers are located in Appendix B.

Respiratory System

http://evolve.elsevier.com/Buck/step

THEORY

Without the use of reference material, complete the following:

Respiratory Terminology

Match the following terms and prefixes to the correct definitions:

1. _____ Polyp
2. _____ Rhino-
3. _____ Endoscopy
4. _____ Sinuses
5. _____ Antrum
6. _____ Antrotomy
7. _____ Laryngo-
8. _____ Bronchoscopy
9. _____ Thoracentesis
10. _____ Thoracotomy
11. _____ Thoracostomy
12. _____ Thoracoscopy
13. _____ Lobectomy
14. _____ Pleura
15. _____ Pneumo-
16. _____ Embolectomy

a. Excision of a lobe of the lung
b. Maxillary sinus
c. Prefix meaning larynx
d. Tumor on a pedicle that bleeds easily and may become malignant
e. Prefix meaning lung or air
f. Surgical puncture of the thoracic cavity, usually using a needle, to remove fluids
g. Inspection of the bronchial tree using a bronchoscope
h. Prefix meaning nose
i. Use of a lighted endoscope to view the pleural spaces and thoracic cavity or perform surgical procedures
j. Removal of blockage (embolism) from vessels
k. Inspection of body organs or cavities using a lighted scope that may be placed through an existing opening or through a small incision
l. Covering of the lungs and thoracic cavity that is moistened with serous fluid to reduce friction during respiratory movements of the lungs
m. Cutting into the thoracic cavity to allow for enlargement of the heart or for drainage
n. Cutting through the antrum wall to make an opening in the sinus
o. Cavities within the nasal bones
p. Surgical incision into the thoracic cavity

Odd-numbered answers are located in Appendix B.

17. What is the name of the item that is placed into the hole in a nasal septum perforation as a repair without surgical grafting?

____

18. What is the name of the surgical procedure for the reshaping of the nose?

____

19. What is the name of the surgical procedure for the rearrangement of the nasal septum often used in patients with a deviated septum?

____

20. This term means destruction by removing, usually by vaporization, chipping, or other erosive process such as laser or cutting:

____

21. Which approach of treating nasal hemorrhage is most difficult to control: posterior or anterior?

____

22. What term describes washing out of an organ?

____

23. What are the two different approaches that can be used to perform a tracheostomy? _______________ and _______________

24. If a surgeon performs a thoracotomy procedure and at the end of the procedure inserts a chest tube for drainage, do you report the insertion of the tube separately? Why?

____

25. If bilateral destruction of maxillary sinuses is performed, what modifier would you use? __________

26. Removal of two lobes of a lung is termed a(n)

____.

Odd-numbered answers are located in Appendix B.

PRACTICAL

With the use of the CPT and ICD-10-CM manuals, complete the following:

27. Endoscopic maxillary antrostomy with removal of granulation tissue.

    CPT Code: ________________

28. Ben is a 5-year-old who swallowed a nickel. Patient needed an indirect laryngoscopy to remove this foreign body.

    CPT Code: ________________

29. Bronchoscopy with transbronchial biopsies of two lobes of the right lung.

    CPT Codes: ________________, ________________

30. Flexible bronchoscopy with brushings.

    CPT Code: ________________

31. Diagnostic flexible fiberoptic laryngoscopy.

    CPT Code: ________________

32. Intranasal biopsy.

    CPT Code: ________________

33. Cauterization of superficial mucosa of bilateral inferior turbinates.

    CPT Code: ________________

34. Primary rhinoplasty with elevation of nasal tip.

    CPT Code: ________________

35. Extensive bilateral removal of nasal polyps, performed in the hospital outpatient department.

    CPT Codes: ________________, ________________

36. Insertion of a septal button.

    CPT Code: ________________

37. Direct operative laryngoscopy with biopsy, with use of the operating microscope.

    CPT Code: ________________

Odd-numbered answers are located in Appendix B.

38. Establishment and subsequent insertion of voice button following construction of a transesophageal fistula.

    CPT Code: ____________________

39. Arytenoidectomy; external approach.

    CPT Code(s): ____________________

40. Laryngoscopy, with stroboscopy.

    CPT Code(s): ____________________

41. Nasotracheal catheter aspiration.

    CPT Code(s): ____________________

42. Cervical tracheoplasty.

    CPT Code(s): ____________________

43. Revision of a tracheostomy scar.

    CPT Code(s): ____________________

44. Thoracentesis for aspiration of the pleural space, without image guidance.

    CPT Code(s): ____________________

45. Surgical thoracoscopy, with removal of a clot from pericardial.

    CPT Code(s): ____________________

46. Double lung transplant with cardiopulmonary bypass.

    CPT Code(s): ____________________

47. Repair hernia of the lung through the chest wall.

    CPT Code(s): ____________________

48. Open closure of a major bronchial fistula.

    CPT Code(s): ____________________

49. Therapeutic fracture of inferior nasal turbinate bone, closed.

    CPT Code(s): ____________________

User to decide number of codes necessary to correctly answer the question.

Odd-numbered answers are located in Appendix B.

50. Sinusotomy, sphenoid, without biopsy for acute sinusitis.

CPT Code(s): ___________________

ICD-10-CM Code(s): _______________

51. Tracheostoma revision, simple, without flap rotation due to infection of tracheostomy by cellulitis.

CPT Code(s): ___________________

ICD-10-CM Code(s): _______________

52. Bronchial biopsy, bronchoscopic, due to chronic cough.

CPT Code(s): ___________________

ICD-10-CM Code(s): _______________

53. Total pneumonectomy due to occupational asbestosis.

CPT Code(s): ___________________

ICD-10-CM Code(s): _______________

54. Diagnostic thoracoscopy of the pericardial sac, with biopsy for chronic rheumatic pericarditis.

CPT Code(s): ___________________

ICD-10-CM Code(s): _______________

55. Extrapleural resection of the ribs, all stages for deformed ribs, congenital.

CPT Code(s): ___________________

ICD-10-CM Code(s): _______________

56. Carinal reconstruction for lung cancer, primary, malignant.

CPT Code(s): ___________________

ICD-10-CM Code(s): _______________

User to decide number of codes necessary to correctly answer the question.

Odd-numbered answers are located in Appendix B.

57. Instillation, via a catheter, of an agent for pleurodesis for malignant pleural effusion due to ovarian cancer.

    CPT Code(s): ____________________

    ICD-10-CM Code(s): ________________

58. Excision of dermoid cyst of the nose, complex.

    CPT Code(s): ____________________

    ICD-10-CM Code(s): ________________

REPORTS

In Appendix A of this workbook you will find a section titled Reports, which contains original reports. Read the reports indicated below and supply the appropriate CPT and ICD-10-CM codes on the following lines:

59. Report 19

    CPT Code(s): ____________________

    ICD-10-CM Code(s): ________________

60. Report 21

    CPT Code(s): ____________________

    ICD-10-CM Code(s): ________________

61. Report 23

    CPT Code(s): ____________________

    ICD-10-CM Code(s): ________________

62. Report 24

    CPT Code(s): ____________________

    ICD-10-CM Code(s): ________________

User to decide number of codes necessary to correctly answer the question.

Odd-numbered answers are located in Appendix B.

Cardiovascular System

http://evolve.elsevier.com/Buck/step

THEORY

Cardiovascular Terminology

Without the use of reference material, match the following terms to the correct definitions:

1. _____ Pericardium
2. _____ Cardiopulmonary
3. _____ Bypass
4. _____ Pacemaker
5. _____ Single-chamber device
6. _____ Dual-chamber device
7. _____ Electrode
8. _____ Ventricle
9. _____ Atrium
10. _____ Implantable defibrillator
11. _____ Artery

a. Lead attached to a generator that carries the electrical current from the generator to the atria or ventricles

b. To go around

c. Surgically placed device that directs an electrical current shock to the heart to restore rhythm

d. Electrode of the pacemaker is placed only in the atrium or only in the ventricle, but not in both places

e. Membranous sac enclosing the heart and ends of the great vessels

f. Vessel that carries oxygenated blood from the heart to the body tissues

g. Refers to the heart and lungs

h. Electrodes of the pacemaker are placed in both the right atrium and the right ventricle of the heart

i. Chamber in the upper part of the heart

j. Electrical device that controls the beating of the heart by electrical impulses

k. Chamber in the lower part of the heart

Odd-numbered answers are located in Appendix B.

Match the following terms to the correct definitions:

12. _____ Vein
13. _____ Aneurysm
14. _____ Embolism
15. _____ Thrombosis
16. _____ Endarterectomy
17. _____ Angioplasty
18. _____ Injection
19. _____ Catheter
20. _____ Arteriovenous fistula
21. _____ Anomaly
22. _____ Ischemia
23. _____ Cardiopulmonary bypass
24. _____ Fistula
25. _____ Shunt

a. Forcing of fluid into a vessel or cavity

b. Blood bypasses the heart through a heart-lung machine during open heart surgery

c. Vessel that carries deoxygenated blood to the heart from the body tissues

d. Blood clot

e. Abnormal opening from one area to another area within the body or to outside of the body

f. Blockage of a blood vessel by a blood clot or other matter that has moved from another area of the body through the circulatory system

g. Direct communication (passage) between an artery and vein

h. Tube placed into the body to put fluid in or take fluid out

i. Surgical or percutaneous procedure on a vessel to dilate the vessel open, used in treatment of atherosclerotic disease

j. A sac of clotted blood or fluid formed in the circulatory system (e.g., vein or artery)

k. Incision into an artery to remove the inner lining to remove disease or blockage

l. Divert or make an artificial passage

m. Deficient blood supply caused by obstruction of the circulatory system

n. Abnormality

26. The term that describes the procedure in which the surgeon withdraws fluid from the pericardial space by means of a needle inserted into the space is ________________.

Odd-numbered answers are located in Appendix B.

27. Codes for excision of cardiac tumors are divided based on whether the tumor is located ________________ or ________________.

28. What are the names of two devices that are inserted into the body to electrically shock the heart into regular rhythm? ________________ and ______________________

29. The two approaches used to insert devices that electrically shock the heart into regular rhythm are ________________ and ________________.

30. If the patient is returned to the operating room for repositioning or replacement of the pacemaker or implantable defibrillator during the global period, modifier __________ would be appended to the code.

31. If a physician implanted a pacemaker and 10 days later the patient returns to the same surgeon for removal of sutures, would you charge for the service? Why or why not?

__________, ____

32. If a patient is seen for a rash on the heel of the foot by the same physician who implanted a pacemaker 20 days earlier, would you bill for the office service for the rash? __________

33. When you bill for E/M services unrelated to a pacemaker implantation during the allowable follow-up days, what modifier would you use on the code to alert the third-party payer? __________

34. What are the four cardiac valves? ________________, ________________, ________________, and ________________

35. What is the name of the device that can be surgically implanted into the subcutaneous tissue in the upper left quadrant to record heart rhythms when the patient depresses a button?

____

36. What arteries feed the heart? __________________________________

37. When a heart artery is clogged and the heart muscle performs at a low level as a result of a lack of blood, the condition is called ________________ ischemia.

Odd-numbered answers are located in Appendix B.

38. When a heart artery is clogged and the heart muscle dies, the condition is called __________________ ischemia.

39. A mass of undissolved matter in the blood that is transported by the blood current is a(n) __________________.

40. Local anesthesia, catheter introduction, and injection of __________________ __________________ are procedures that are included in a vascular injection.

PRACTICAL

Using the CPT and ICD-10-CM manuals, code the following:

41. Valvuloplasty of the aortic valve using transventricular dilation with cardiopulmonary bypass.

    CPT Code: __________________

42. Replacement aortic valve, with cardiopulmonary bypass, with prosthetic valve.

    CPT Code: __________________

43. Valvuloplasty, tricuspid valve, with ring insertion.

    CPT Code: __________________

44. Repair of a coronary arteriovenous fistula, without cardiopulmonary bypass.

    CPT Code: __________________

45. Routine ECG with 12 leads, with both the professional and technical components.

    CPT Code: __________________

46. External electrical cardioversion.

    CPT Code: __________________

47. Percutaneous balloon angioplasty; one coronary vessel.

    CPT Code: __________________

48. CPR (Cardiopulmonary resuscitation).

    CPT Code: __________________

Odd-numbered answers are located in Appendix B.

49. Electrocardiogram with interpretation and report only.

    CPT Code: ___________________

50. Bypass graft of the common carotid-ipsilateral internal carotid artery using synthetic vein.

    CPT Code: ___________________

51. Ligation of temporal artery.

    CPT Code: ___________________

52. Ligation of a common iliac vein.

    CPT Code: ___________________

53. Open transluminal balloon angioplasty aorta.

    CPT Code: ___________________

54. Coronary artery bypass, single artery, for coronary atherosclerosis of native coronary artery in a transplanted heart.

    CPT Code: ___________________

    ICD-10-CM Code: _______________

55. Coronary artery bypass, four veins, no arteries. Diagnosis of acute coronary insufficiency.

    CPT Code(s): ___________________

    ICD-10-CM Code(s): _______________

56. Repair of injury to intra-abdominal blood vessel, inferior vena cava, hepatic vein, with a vein graft.

    CPT Code(s): ___________________

    ICD-10-CM Code(s): _______________

57. Percutaneous insertion of an intra-aortic balloon assist device due to initial episode of acute myocardial infarction and cardiogenic shock.

    CPT Code(s): ___________________

    ICD-10-CM Code(s): _______________

User to decide number of codes necessary to correctly answer the question.

Odd-numbered answers are located in Appendix B.

58. Repair of a traumatic arteriovenous fistula of a lower extremity.

CPT Code(s): ___________________

ICD-10-CM Code(s): _______________

59. Repair of congenital atrial septal defect, secundum, with bypass and patch.

CPT Code(s): ___________________

ICD-10-CM Code(s): _______________

60. Repair of a patent ductus arteriosus by division on a 16-year-old patient.

CPT Code(s): ___________________

ICD-10-CM Code(s): _______________

61. Reoperation of one arterial coronary bypass graft and one vein bypass graft for arteriosclerosis of native arteries, 3 months following the initial procedure.

CPT Code(s): ___________________

ICD-10-CM Code(s): _______________

REPORTS

In Appendix A of this workbook you will find a section titled Reports, which contains original reports. Read the reports indicated below and supply the appropriate CPT and ICD-10-CM codes on the following lines:

62. Report 25

CPT Code(s): ___________________

ICD-10-CM Code(s): _______________

63. Report 26

CPT Code(s): ___________________

ICD-10-CM Code(s): _______________

64. Report 27

CPT Code(s): ___________________

ICD-10-CM Code(s): _______________

User to decide number of codes necessary to correctly answer the question.

Odd-numbered answers are located in Appendix B.

65. Report 96

CPT Code(s): ____________________

ICD-10-CM Code(s): ________________

66. Report 97

CPT Code(s): ____________________

ICD-10-CM Code(s): ________________

User to decide number of codes necessary to correctly answer the question.

Odd-numbered answers are located in Appendix B.

CHAPTER 18

Hemic, Lymphatic, Mediastinum, and Diaphragm

http://evolve.elsevier.com/Buck/step

THEORY

Hemic and Lymphatic Terminology

Without the use of reference material, match the following terms to the correct definitions:

1. _____ Axillary nodes
2. _____ Splenectomy
3. _____ Splenoportography
4. _____ Allogenic
5. _____ Thoracic duct
6. _____ Retroperitoneal
7. _____ Jugular nodes
8. _____ Cystic hygroma
9. _____ Cloquet's node
10. _____ Inguinofemoral
11. _____ Cannulation
12. _____ Abscess

a. Behind the sac holding the abdominal organs and viscera (peritoneum)
b. Excision of the spleen
c. Insertion of a tube into a duct or cavity
d. Lymph nodes located next to the large vein in the neck
e. Radiographic procedure to allow visualization of the splenic and portal veins of the spleen
f. Of the same species, but genetically different
g. Collection and distribution point for lymph and the largest lymph vessel located in the chest
h. Congenital deformity or benign tumor of the lymphatic system
i. Also called a gland; it is the highest of the deep groin lymph nodes
j. Term that refers to the groin and thigh
k. Lymph nodes located in the armpit
l. Localization of pus

Odd-numbered answers are located in Appendix B.

Match the following terms to the correct definitions:

13. _____ Autologous, autogenous
14. _____ Aspiration
15. _____ Stem cell
16. _____ Transplantation
17. _____ Lymph node
18. _____ Lymphadenitis
19. _____ Lymphangiotomy
20. _____ Lymphadenectomy

a. Grafting of tissue from one source to another
b. Immature blood cells
c. Incision into a lymphatic vessel
d. Inflammation of a lymph node
e. Excision of a lymph node (or nodes)
f. From oneself
g. Use of a needle and syringe to withdraw fluid
h. Station along the lymphatic system

Mediastinum and Diaphragm Terminology

Match the following terms to the correct definitions:

21. _____ Mediastinum
22. _____ Diaphragm
23. _____ Mediastinotomy
24. _____ Fundoplasty
25. _____ Pyloroplasty
26. _____ Diaphragmatic hernia
27. _____ Mediastinoscopy
28. _____ Imbrication
29. _____ Transthoracic
30. _____ Transabdominal
31. _____ Paraesophageal hiatus hernia
32. _____ Gastroplasty
33. _____ Vagotomy

a. Overlapping
b. Surgical separation of the vagus nerve
c. Muscular wall that separates the thoracic and abdominal cavities
d. Incision and repair of the pyloric channel
e. Operation on the stomach for repair or reconfiguration
f. Repair of the bottom of an organ or muscle
g. Hernia that is near the esophagus
h. Hernia of the diaphragm
i. Across the abdomen
j. Cutting into the mediastinum
k. Across the thorax
l. Use of an endoscope inserted through a small incision to view the mediastinum
m. The area between the lungs that contains the heart, aorta, trachea, lymph nodes, thymus gland, esophagus, and bronchial tubes

Odd-numbered answers are located in Appendix B.

PRACTICAL

Using the CPT and ICD-10-CM manuals, code the following:

34. Injection procedure for identification of the sentinel node with intradermal radioisotope injection for the staging of clinically negative axillae in a patient with primary malignant neoplasm of the central portion of the right breast.

    CPT Code(s): ____________________

    ICD-10-CM Code(s): ________________

35. Radical cervical lymphadenectomy for patient with malignant primary cancer of the nipple of the left breast. Pathology findings of the lymphadenectomy were positive.

    CPT Code(s): ____________________

    ICD-10-CM Code(s): ________________

36. Drainage of an extensive lymph node abscess. Pathology report indicated *Staphylococcus*.

    CPT Code(s): ____________________

    ICD-10-CM Code(s): ________________

37. Autologous bone marrow transplantation for a patient who has acute myelogenous leukemia that has not shown any signs of remission.

    CPT Code(s): ____________________

    ICD-10-CM Code(s): ________________

38. Partial splenectomy for a 3-year-old child with sickle cell disease, Hb-C with crisis.

    CPT Code: ____________________

    ICD-10-CM Code: ________________

39. Harvesting of bone marrow for transplantation from a father for subsequent transplantation into the daughter. Report only the harvesting service.

    CPT Code: ____________________

    ICD-10-CM Code: ________________

User to decide number of codes necessary to correctly answer the question.

Odd-numbered answers are located in Appendix B.

40. Repair of laceration of diaphragm by means of abdominal approach.

    CPT Code: ___________________

41. Excision of mediastinal cyst.

    CPT Code: ___________________

42. Resection of diaphragm with simple repair.

    CPT Code: ___________________

43. Preparation of stem (hematopoietic progenitor) cells for transplantation that included thawing of previously frozen cells and washing of the cells.

    CPT Code: ___________________

44. Laparoscopic removal of the spleen.

    CPT Code: ___________________

45. A radiologist performs lymphoscintigraphy in the radiology department. A few hours later, the patient is taken to the operating room where the general surgeon injects blue dye into the internal mammary lymph node and then excises a sentinel lymph node.

    CPT Codes: ___________________-26 (for performing both the injection and imaging of the radioisotope in the radiology department [nuclear medicine, lymph nodes]), ___________________-59 (for injecting the blue dye), and ___________________ (for excision of the sentinel lymph node in the operating room)

REPORT

In Appendix A of this workbook you will find a section titled Reports, which contains original reports. Read the report indicated below and supply the appropriate CPT and ICD-10-CM codes on the following lines:

46. Report 89

    CPT Code: ___________________

    ICD-10-CM Codes: _______________,

    _______________ (External Cause code for how accident occurred),

    ___________________ (Y code)

Odd-numbered answers are located in Appendix B.

Digestive System

http://evolve.elsevier.com/Buck/step

THEORY

Digestive Terminology

Without the use of reference material, match the following terms to the correct definitions:

1. _____ Gloss-
2. _____ Gastro-
3. _____ Anastomosis
4. _____ Hernia
5. _____ Gastrointestinal
6. _____ Ostomy
7. _____ Colostomy
8. _____ Ileostomy
9. _____ Jejunostomy

a. Artificial opening between the colon and the abdominal wall

b. Prefix meaning tongue

c. Organ or tissue protruding through the wall or cavity that usually contains it

d. Combining form meaning stomach

e. Artificial opening between the ileum and the abdominal wall

f. Surgical connection of two tubular structures, such as two pieces of the intestine

g. Pertaining to the stomach and intestine

h. Artificial opening

i. Artificial opening between the jejunum and the abdominal wall

Odd-numbered answers are located in Appendix B.

Without reference material, match the following terms to the correct definitions:

10. _____ Gastrostomy
11. _____ Proctosigmoidoscopy
12. _____ Sigmoidoscopy
13. _____ Colonoscopy
14. _____ Cholangiography
15. _____ Chole-
16. _____ Hepat-
17. _____ Incarcerated
18. _____ Reducible

a. Regarding hernias, a constricted, irreducible hernia that may cause obstruction of an intestine

b. Artificial opening between the stomach and the abdominal wall

c. Radiographic recording of the bile ducts

d. Able to be corrected or put back into a normal position

e. Endoscopic examination of the entire colon that may include part of the terminal ileum

f. Combining form meaning liver

g. Endoscopic examination of the entire rectum and sigmoid colon that may include a portion of the descending colon

h. Combining form meaning bile

i. Endoscopic examination of the sigmoid colon and rectum

PRACTICAL

Using the CPT and ICD-10-CM manuals, code the following:

19. Rigid esophagoscopy with removal of a foreign body.

    CPT Code: ________________

20. Ligation of an intraoral salivary duct.

    CPT Code: ________________

21. Cervical approach for suture of an esophageal wound.

    CPT Code: ________________

22. Enterotomy of the small intestine for removal of a foreign body.

    CPT Code: ________________

Odd-numbered answers are located in Appendix B.

23. Complicated revision of a colostomy.

    CPT Code: __________________

24. Frenotomy, labial.

    CPT Code: __________________

25. Excision of a palate lesion without closure.

    CPT Code: __________________

26. Removal of a foreign body from the pharynx.

    CPT Code: __________________

27. Amy is an 18-year-old with severe snoring. She is having an adenoidectomy in order to treat her snoring.

    CPT Code: __________________

28. Partial colectomy with colostomy.

    CPT Code: __________________

29. Open repair of an incarcerated recurrent inguinal hernia.

    CPT Code: __________________

30. Surgical laparoscopic placement of a gastric band.

    CPT Code: __________________

31. Full-thickness repair of the vermilion of the lip.

    CPT Code: __________________

32. Simple repair of 1.6-cm laceration of floor of mouth.

    CPT Code: __________________

33. Bilateral parotid duct diversion.

    CPT Code: __________________

34. Surgical laparoscopic repair of a paraesophageal hernia with fundoplasty with implantation of mesh.

    CPT Code: __________________

Odd-numbered answers are located in Appendix B.

35. Biopsy of the stomach by laparotomy.

    CPT Code: ________________

36. Nontube open ileostomy.

    CPT Code: ________________

37. Colorrhaphy for multiple perforations of large intestine sustained in auto accident. No colostomy was required.

    CPT Code: ________________

38. Incision and drainage of perirectal abscess.

    CPT Code: ________________

39. Diagnostic abdominal laparoscopy.

    CPT Code: ________________

40. PREPROCEDURE DIAGNOSIS: Screening colonoscopy.

    POSTPROCEDURE DIAGNOSIS: Colon polyps.

    PREMEDICATIONS: Fentanyl 100 mcg and Versed 4 mg.

    PROCEDURE: A colonoscopy was performed to the cecum. The scope was advanced to the cecum under direct vision without any difficulty.

    FINDINGS: The cecum, ascending, transverse, descending, and sigmoid colon were normal. In the descending colon, there was a 2-mm polyp that was biopsied and submitted for histology.

    ASSESSMENT: Diminutive colon polyps.

    Pathology Report later indicated benign polyps.

    CPT Code: ________________

    ICD-10-CM Codes: ______________

41. The patient presented to the emergency department complaining of vomiting coffee-ground material several times within the past 2 hours. He has abdominal pain and has been unable to eat for the past 24 hours. He is dizzy and light-headed. Two stools today have been black and tarry. While in the emergency department, he vomited bright-red blood and some coffee-ground material. A nasogastric tube was inserted and attached to suction with fluoroscopy. An abdominal exam showed a fluid wave consistent with ascites. An IV of lactated ringers was started, and CBC and clotting studies were drawn. A high-complexity medical decision making was documented. A GI consultant

Odd-numbered answers are located in Appendix B.

was called and the patient was taken to Endoscopy for further evaluation of upper GI bleeding. Diagnosis: hematemesis, rule out esophageal varices; blood loss anemia (CBC review) acute; ascites. Code the services of the ED physician.

CPT Codes: ________________, ________________

ICD-10-CM Codes: ______________, ______________, ______________

REPORTS

In Appendix A of this workbook you will find a section titled Reports, which contains original reports. Read the reports indicated below and supply the appropriate CPT and ICD-10-CM codes on the following lines:

42. Report 22

    CPT Code(s): ________________

    ICD-10-CM Code(s): ______________

43. Report 31

    CPT Code(s): ________________

    ICD-10-CM Code(s): ______________

44. Report 32

    CPT Code(s): ________________

    ICD-10-CM Code(s): ______________

45. Report 33

    CPT Code(s): ________________

    ICD-10-CM Code(s): ______________

46. Report 34

    CPT Code(s): ________________

    ICD-10-CM Code(s): ______________

47. Report 35

    CPT Code(s): ________________

    ICD-10-CM Code(s): ______________

User to decide number of codes necessary to correctly answer the question.

Odd-numbered answers are located in Appendix B.

48. Report 39

CPT Code(s): ____________________

ICD-10-CM Code(s): ________________

49. Report 98

CPT Code(s): ____________________

ICD-10-CM Code(s): ________________

User to decide number of codes necessary to correctly answer the question.

Odd-numbered answers are located in Appendix B.

Urinary and Male Genital Systems

http://evolve.elsevier.com/Buck/step

THEORY

Urinary System Terminology

Without the use of reference material, match the following terms to the correct definitions:

1. _____ Calculus/calculi
2. _____ Cystolithectomy
3. _____ Cystometrogram (CMG)
4. _____ Endopyelotomy
5. _____ Exstrophy
6. _____ Nephrectomy
7. _____ Fulguration
8. _____ Kock pouch
9. _____ Lithotripsy
10. _____ Marsupialization
11. _____ Nephro-
12. _____ Nephrostomy

a. With the use of an endoscope, an incision is made to correct stenosis of the ureteropelvic junction

b. Kidney removal

c. Crushing of a gallbladder or urinary bladder stone followed by irrigation to wash the fragment out

d. A concretion of mineral salts, also called a stone

e. Surgical creation of a urinary bladder from a segment of the ileum

f. Condition in which an organ is turned inside out

g. Measurement of the pressures and capacity of the urinary bladder

h. Creation of a channel into the renal pelvis of the kidney

i. Surgical procedure that creates an open pouch from an internal abscess

j. Removal of a calculus from the urinary bladder

k. Use of electrical current to destroy tissue

l. Prefix meaning kidney

Odd-numbered answers are located in Appendix B.

Without the use of reference material, match the following terms to the correct definitions:

13. _____ Perivesical
14. _____ Perirenal
15. _____ Pyelo-
16. _____ Pyeloplasty
17. _____ Pyelostomy
18. _____ Renal pelvis
19. _____ Retroperitoneal
20. _____ Transureteroureterostomy
21. _____ Ureterolithotomy
22. _____ Ureterotomy
23. _____ Urethrocystography
24. _____ Urethrorrhaphy

a. Prefix meaning renal pelvis
b. Removal of a stone from the ureter
c. Surgical connection of one ureter to the other ureter
d. Surgical creation of an opening into the renal pelvis
e. Suturing of the urethra
f. Behind the sac holding the abdominal organs and viscera (peritoneum)
g. Around the kidney
h. Radiography of the bladder and urethra
i. Around the bladder
j. Funnel-shaped sac in the kidney where urine is received
k. Surgical reconstruction of the renal pelvis
l. Incision into the ureter

Male Genital Terminology

Without the use of reference material, match the following terms to the correct definitions:

25. _____ Cavernosa-saphenous
26. _____ Orchiectomy
27. _____ Hydrocele
28. _____ Vasogram
29. _____ Varicocele
30. _____ Vas deferens

a. Tube that carries sperm from the epididymis to the urethra
b. Swelling of a scrotal vein
c. Creation of a connection between the cavity of the penis and a vein
d. Castration
e. Sac of fluid
f. Recording of the flow in the vas deferens

Odd-numbered answers are located in Appendix B.

Without reference material, match the following terms to the correct definitions:

31. _____ Electrodesiccation
32. _____ Corpora cavernosa
33. _____ Epididymis
34. _____ Cavernosography
35. _____ Cavernosometry
36. _____ Plethysmography
37. _____ Hypospadias
38. _____ Vesiculectomy
39. _____ Prostatotomy

a. Excision of a seminal vesicle
b. Determining the changes in volume of an organ part or body
c. Incision into the prostate
d. Destruction of a lesion by the use of electrical current radiated through a needle
e. A tube located on the top of the testes that stores sperm
f. Measurements of the pressure in a cavity (e.g., penis)
g. Two cavities of the penis
h. Radiographic measurement of a cavity (e.g., the main part of the penis)
i. Congenital deformity of the urethra in which the urethral opening is on the underside of the penis rather than on the end

Without reference material, match the following terms to the correct definitions:

40. _____ Lymphadenectomy
41. _____ Priapism
42. _____ Chordee
43. _____ Urethroplasty
44. _____ Penoscrotal
45. _____ Spermatocele

a. Surgical repair of the urethra
b. Referring to the penis and scrotum
c. Painful condition in which the penis is constantly erect
d. Excision of lymph node(s)
e. Condition resulting in the penis being bent downward
f. Cyst filled with spermatozoa

Odd-numbered answers are located in Appendix B.

Without reference material, match the following terms to the correct definitions:

46. _____ Tumescence
47. _____ Cavernosa-corpus spongiosum shunt
48. _____ Cavernosa-glans penis fistulization
49. _____ Orchiopexy
50. _____ Vasovasostomy
51. _____ Vasovasorrhaphy

a. Creation of a connection between a cavity of the penis and the urethra
b. Creation of a connection between a cavity of the penis and the glans penis, which overlaps the penis cavity
c. Reversal of a vasectomy
d. Surgical procedure to release undescended testis
e. Suturing of the vas deferens
f. State of being swollen

Without reference material, match the following terms to the correct definitions:

52. _____ Epididymectomy
53. _____ Epididymovasostomy
54. _____ Vasotomy
55. _____ Vesiculotomy
56. _____ Seminal vesicle
57. _____ Tunica vaginalis

a. Creation of a new connection between the vas deferens and epididymis
b. Incision in the vas deferens
c. Covering of the testes
d. Incision into the seminal vesicle
e. Gland that secretes fluid that ultimately becomes semen
f. Surgical removal of the epididymis

PRACTICAL

Using the CPT and ICD-10-CM manuals, code the following:

58. Endoscopy for resection of primary malignant renal pelvis tumor through an established stoma.

    CPT Code:__________________

    ICD-10-CM Code: _______________

59. Aspiration of a solitary, non-congenital renal cyst through percutaneous needle.

    CPT Code: __________________

    ICD-10-CM Code: _______________

Odd-numbered answers are located in Appendix B.

60. Ureteroureterostomy performed for urinary tract obstruction.

    CPT Code: ________________

    ICD-10-CM Code: ____________

61. Transurethral incision of the prostate to treat benign hypertrophic prostatitis.

    CPT Code: ________________

    ICD-10-CM Code: ____________

62. Cystourethroscopy due to intermittent hematuria.

    CPT Code: ________________

    ICD-10-CM Code: ____________

63. Abdominal orchiopexy to release undescended intra-abdominal testes.

    CPT Code: ________________

    ICD-10-CM Code: ____________

64. Complicated prostatotomy of prostate cyst.

    CPT Code: ________________

    ICD-10-CM Code: ____________

65. Closure of nephrocutaneous fistula.

    CPT Code: ________________

66. A steroid injection for urethral stricture using a cystourethroscope.

    CPT Code(s): ________________

67. Total urethrectomy of a 44-year-old male.

    CPT Code(s): ________________

68. Circumcision using clamp, routine.

    CPT Code(s): ________________

    ICD-10-CM Code(s): ____________

User to decide number of codes necessary to correctly answer the question.

Odd-numbered answers are located in Appendix B.

69. Excision of Skene's glands.

    CPT Code(s): ____________________

70. Bilateral shunt of corpora cavernosa–saphenous vein for priapism.

    CPT Code(s): ____________________

71. Vasovasorrhaphy.

    CPT Code(s): ____________________

72. Exposure of the prostate for insertion of radioactive substance.

    CPT Code(s): ____________________

73. Surgical reduction of torsion of testis with fixation of contralateral testis.

    CPT Code(s): ____________________

74. Distal hypospadias repair with chordee using a V-flap advancement, completed in one stage.

    CPT Code(s): ____________________

75. Simple destruction of four lesions of the penis using cryosurgery.

    CPT Code(s): ____________________

76. Repair of an incomplete circumcision.

    CPT Code(s): ____________________

77. Drainage of a scrotal wall abscess.

    CPT Code(s): ____________________

78. Ureterectomy, with repair of the bladder cuff.

    CPT Code(s): ____________________

REPORTS

In Appendix A of this workbook you will find a section titled Reports, which contains original reports. Read the reports indicated below and supply the appropriate CPT and ICD-10-CM codes on the following lines:

79. Report 36

    CPT Code(s): ____________________

User to decide number of codes necessary to correctly answer the question.

Odd-numbered answers are located in Appendix B.

80. Report 37

 CPT Code(s): ________________

 ICD-10-CM Code(s): ____________

81. Report 38

 CPT Code(s): ________________

 ICD-10-CM Code(s): ____________

82. Report 81

 CPT Code(s): ________________

83. Report 82

 CPT Code(s): ________________

84. Report 83

 CPT Code(s): ________________

 ICD-10-CM Code(s): ____________

85. Report 84

 CPT Code(s): ________________

86. Report 99

 CPT Code(s): ________________

 ICD-10-CM Code(s): ____________

User to decide number of codes necessary to correctly answer the question.

Odd-numbered answers are located in Appendix B.

CHAPTER 21

Reproductive, Intersex Surgery, Female Genital System, and Maternity Care and Delivery

http://evolve.elsevier.com/Buck/step

THEORY

Female Genital Terminology

Without the use of reference material, match the following terms to the correct definitions:

1. _____ Vulva
2. _____ Perineum
3. _____ Introitus
4. _____ Vagina
5. _____ Cervix uteri
6. _____ Corpus uteri
7. _____ Oviduct
8. _____ Salpingo-
9. _____ Oophor-
10. _____ Curettage
11. _____ Dilation
12. _____ Cystocele
13. _____ Rectocele

a. Herniation of the bladder into the vagina
b. Rounded, cone-shaped neck of the uterus, part of it protruding into the vagina
c. Prefix meaning ovary
d. External female genitalia, including labia majora, labia minora, clitoris, and vaginal opening
e. Uterus
f. Herniation of the rectal wall through the posterior wall of the vagina
g. Prefix meaning tube
h. Opening or entrance to the vagina
i. Scraping of a cavity using a spoon-shaped instrument
j. Expansion
k. Area between the vulva and anus
l. Canal from the external female genitalia to the uterus
m. Fallopian tube

Odd-numbered answers are located in Appendix B.

Maternity Care and Delivery Terminology

Without the use of reference material, match the following terms to the correct definitions:

14. _____ Antepartum
15. _____ Postpartum
16. _____ Abortion
17. _____ Delivery
18. _____ Cesarean
19. _____ Ectopic
20. _____ Version
21. _____ Amniocentesis
22. _____ Cordocentesis
23. _____ Chorionic villus sampling (CVS)
24. _____ Hysterotomy
25. _____ Salpingectomy
26. _____ Oophorectomy
27. _____ Hysterectomy
28. _____ Hysterorrhaphy
29. _____ Tocolysis
30. _____ VBAC

a. Turning of the fetus from a presentation other than cephalic (head down) to cephalic for ease of birth
b. Termination of pregnancy
c. Surgical opening through abdominal wall for delivery
d. Before childbirth
e. After childbirth
f. Pregnancy outside the uterus (e.g., in the fallopian tube)
g. Childbirth
h. Incision into the uterus
i. Surgical removal of the uterus
j. Percutaneous aspiration of amniotic fluid
k. Surgical removal of ovary
l. Biopsy of the outermost part of the placenta
m. Suturing of the uterus
n. Repression of uterine contractions
o. Surgical removal of a fallopian tube
p. Vaginal delivery after previous cesarean delivery
q. Procedure to obtain a fetal blood sample, also called a percutaneous umbilical blood sampling

Odd-numbered answers are located in Appendix B.

Without the use of reference material, answer the following:

31. Plastic repair of the __________________ is surgical repair of the opening to the vagina.

32. An incision into the vagina to gain access to the pelvic cavity is __________________.

33. The insertion of a long needle into the back wall of the vagina to gain access to a peritoneal cul de sac abscess is __________________.

34. A vaginal support device is a(n) __________________.

35. When reporting the service of the introduction of a diaphragm, the cost of the diaphragm is included in the introduction.

    True or False? ___________

36. The term that describes the procedure in which the surgeon strengthens the wall of the weakened vagina by pulling together the weakened vaginal area with sutures is:

    ____

37. The microscope that is used to view the vagina is a(n) __________________.

38. The services described in the Manipulation category of the Vagina subheading require this type of anesthesia: __________________

39. LEEP means ____.

40. Endometrial __________________ is a biopsy of the mucous lining of the uterus.

41. What one procedure represents the majority of the codes in the Corpus Uteri subheading? __________________

42. Hydatidiform mole, also known as a "molar pregnancy," results from genetic abnormalities.

    True or False? ___________

43. A hysterosalpingography would have a component code from what section of the CPT manual? __________________

Odd-numbered answers are located in Appendix B.

44. The first rule of a laparoscopy is that a surgical laparoscopy always includes this type of laparoscopy: ________________

45. In what subheading would you find the codes to report fallopian tube services?

____

46. The three methods of tubal ligation are ligation, ________________, and ________________.

47. Gestation is divided into three time periods that are termed ________________.

48. The first gestation time period is LMP to less than __________ weeks 0 days, the second is __________ weeks 0 days to less than __________ weeks 0 days, and the third is __________ weeks 0 days until delivery.

49. What does EDD stand for?

________________ ________________ of ________________

50. Preparation of the cervix for birth or dilation is termed cervical ________________.

51. If a physician other than the attending provided only one office visit to a patient before delivery, a code from what section of the CPT manual would be used to report this service? ________________

52. The time after delivery is referred to as ________________.

PRACTICAL

Using the CPT manual, code the following:

53. Dilation of the vagina under anesthesia.

CPT Code: ________________

54. Plastic repair of a urethrocele.

CPT Code: ________________

Odd-numbered answers are located in Appendix B.

55. Labial adhesions lysis.

    CPT Code: ________________

56. Simple complete vulvectomy.

    CPT Code: ________________

57. Surgical hysteroscopy with polypectomy and dilation and curettage.

    CPT Code: ________________

58. Transposition of the left ovary.

    CPT Code: ________________

59. Bilateral wedge resection of ovaries.

    CPT Code: ________________

60. Therapeutic amniocentesis with amniotic fluid reduction.

    CPT Code: ________________

61. Drainage of a cyst of the left ovary using the vaginal approach.

    CPT Code(s): ________________

62. Surgical treatment of a second-trimester missed abortion.

    CPT Code(s): ________________

63. Cesarean delivery only.

    CPT Code(s): ________________

64. Hysterorrhaphy of a ruptured, pregnant uterus.

    CPT Code(s): ________________

65. Fetal contraction stress tests, antepartum.

    CPT Code(s): ________________

66. Radical vaginal hysterectomy.

    CPT Code(s): ________________

67. Marsupialization of Bartholin's gland cyst.

    CPT Code(s): ________________

User to decide number of codes necessary to correctly answer the question.

Odd-numbered answers are located in Appendix B.

68. Excision of Bartholin's gland.

    CPT Code(s): ___________________

69. Destruction of extensive vaginal lesions.

    CPT Code(s): ___________________

REPORTS

In Appendix A of this workbook you will find a section titled Reports, which contains original reports. Code only the primary surgery. Read the reports indicated below and supply the appropriate CPT and ICD-10-CM codes on the following lines:

70. Report 20

    CPT Code(s): ___________________

    ICD-10-CM Code(s): _______________

71. Report 28

    CPT Code(s): ___________________

    ICD-10-CM Code(s): _______________

72. Report 29

    CPT Code(s): ___________________

    ICD-10-CM Code(s): _______________

73. Report 30

    CPT Code(s): ___________________

    ICD-10-CM Code(s): _______________

User to decide number of codes necessary to correctly answer the question.

Odd-numbered answers are located in Appendix B.

CHAPTER 22

Endocrine and Nervous Systems

http://evolve.elsevier.com/Buck/step

THEORY

Endocrine System Terminology

Match the following terms to the correct definitions:

1. _____ Isthmus
2. _____ Isthmus, thyroid
3. _____ Isthmusectomy
4. _____ Contralateral
5. _____ Thyroidectomy
6. _____ Thyroglossal duct
7. _____ Thymectomy
8. _____ Adrenal
9. _____ Thyroid
10. _____ Thymus
11. _____ Parathyroid

a. Glands located on the top of the kidneys that produce steroid hormones
b. Produces a hormone to mobilize calcium from the bones to the blood
c. Connection of two regions or structures
d. Surgical removal of the thyroid
e. Produces hormones important to the immune response
f. Surgical removal of the isthmus
g. Surgical removal of the thymus
h. Part of the endocrine system, a gland that produces hormones that regulate metabolism
i. Tissue connection between right and left thyroid lobes
j. Develops in the embryo stage after the formation of the thyroid gland
k. Affecting the opposite side

Odd-numbered answers are located in Appendix B.

Nervous System Terminology

Match the following terms to the correct definitions:

12. _____ Cranium
13. _____ Skull
14. _____ Stereotaxis
15. _____ Laminectomy
16. _____ Somatic nerve
17. _____ Sympathetic nerve
18. _____ Peripheral nerves
19. _____ Shunt
20. _____ Central nervous system

a. A method of identifying a specific area or point in the brain
b. Part of the peripheral nervous system that controls automatic body function; activated under stress
c. That part of the skeleton that encloses the brain
d. Divert or make an artificial passage
e. Twelve pairs of cranial nerves, 31 pairs of spinal nerves, and autonomic nervous system; connects peripheral receptors to the brain and spinal cord
f. Sensory or motor nerve
g. Entire skeletal framework of the head
h. Surgical excision of the lamina
i. Brain and spinal cord

PRACTICAL

Using the CPT manual, code the following:

21. Incision and drainage of an infected thyroglossal duct cyst.

    CPT Code(s): ____________________

22. Removal of a complete cerebrospinal fluid shunt system; without replacement.

    CPT Code(s): ____________________

23. Suture of the posterior tibial nerve.

    CPT Code(s): ____________________

24. Lumbar sympathetic block (left).

    CPT Code: ____________________

25. Microdissection, microrepair ulnar digital nerve left middle finger.

    CPT Codes: ____________________, ____________________

User to decide number of codes necessary to correctly answer the question.

Odd-numbered answers are located in Appendix B.

26. Placement of a dorsal column stimulator with implanted pulse generator, with stereotactic stimulation of spinal cord and pocket creation with connection.

    CPT Code: ___________________

27. Epidural injection of a steroid, caudal.

    CPT Code: ___________________

28. Craniotomy for drainage of an intracranial abscess; infratentorial.

    CPT Code: ___________________

29. Re-operation, skull base surgery, repair of dura mater due to leak of CSF of middle cranial fossa; myocutaneous flap graft.

    CPT Code: ___________________

30. Insertion of a cerebrospinal fluid ventriculoperitoneal shunt for hydrocephalus.

    CPT Code: ___________________

31. Hemilaminectomy, posterior approach, with decompression of two nerve roots and with excision of herniated disc at L1-L2 and foraminotomy at L2-L3.

    CPT Codes: ___________________, ___________________

REPORTS

In Appendix A of this workbook you will find a section titled Reports, which contains original reports. Read the reports indicated below and supply the appropriate CPT and ICD-10-CM codes on the following lines:

32. Report 41

    CPT Codes: ___________________ (arthrodesis with discectomy),

    ___________________ (arthrodesis with discectomy), ___________________

    (instrumentation), ___________________ (allograft),

    ___________________ (evoked potential)

    ICD-10-CM Code: _______________

33. Report 43

    Code(s): ___________________

    ICD-10-CM Code(s): _______________

User to decide number of codes necessary to correctly answer the question.

Odd-numbered answers are located in Appendix B.

CHAPTER 23

Eye, Ocular Adnexa, Auditory, and Operating Microscope

http://evolve.elsevier.com/Buck/step

THEORY

Eye and Ocular Adnexa Terminology

Match the following terms to the correct definitions:

1. _____ Keratoplasty
2. _____ Evisceration
3. _____ Enucleation
4. _____ Exenteration
5. _____ Cataract
6. _____ Sclera
7. _____ Conjunctiva
8. _____ Uveal
9. _____ Tarsorrhaphy
10. _____ Ocular adnexa

a. Surgical repair of the cornea
b. Removal of an eye
c. Opaque covering on or in the lens
d. Lining of the eyelids and covering of the sclera
e. Removal of an organ all in one piece
f. Pulling the viscera outside the body through an incision
g. White outer portion of the eyeball
h. Vascular tissue of the choroids, ciliary body, and iris
i. Suturing together of the eyelids
j. Orbit, extraocular muscles, and eyelid

Odd-numbered answers are located in Appendix B.

Match the following terms to the correct definitions:

11. _____ Anterior segment
12. _____ Posterior segment
13. _____ Blephar/o-
14. _____ Cor/o-
15. _____ Cyclo/o-
16. _____ Dacry/o-
17. _____ Kerat/o-
18. _____ Ocul/o-
19. _____ Dacryocyst/o-
20. _____ Vitre/o-
21. _____ Astigmatism
22. _____ Strabismus

a. Prefix meaning eye

b. Prefix meaning tear/tear duct

c. Parts of the eye located behind the lens

d. Prefix meaning cornea

e. Prefix meaning pertaining to the vitreous body of the eye

f. Prefix meaning ciliary body or eye muscle

g. Parts of the eye in the front of and including the lens, orbit, extraocular muscles, and eyelid

h. Prefix meaning pertaining to the lacrimal sac

i. Extraocular muscle deviation resulting in unequal visual axes

j. Condition in which the refractive surfaces of the eyes are unequal

k. Prefix meaning eyelid

l. Prefix meaning pupil

Odd-numbered answers are located in Appendix B.

Auditory System Terminology

Match the following terms to the correct definitions:

23. _____ Aural atresia
24. _____ Transmastoid antrostomy
25. _____ Labyrinth
26. _____ Tympanic neurectomy
27. _____ Fenestration
28. _____ Parts of the external ear
29. _____ Parts of the middle ear
30. _____ Parts of the inner ear
31. _____ Mastoid-
32. _____ Myring-
33. _____ Audi-
34. _____ Exostosis
35. _____ Oto-
36. _____ Salping(o)-
37. _____ Apicectomy

a. Prefix meaning hearing
b. Auricle, pinna, external acoustic, and meatus
c. Prefix meaning ear
d. Prefix meaning (eustachian) tube
e. Vestibule, semicircular canals, and cochlea
f. Excision of the tympanic nerve
g. Congenital absence of the external auditory canal
h. Creation of a new opening (e.g., on the inner wall of the middle ear)
i. Malleus, incus, and stapes
j. A bony growth
k. Prefix meaning posterior temporal bone
l. Excision of a portion of the temporal bone
m. Called a simple mastoidectomy, it creates an opening in the mastoid for drainage
n. Inner connecting cavities, such as the internal ear
o. Prefix meaning eardrum

PRACTICAL

Using the CPT and ICD-10-CM manuals, code the following:

38. Incision and drainage of conjunctival cysts of left and right eyes.

    CPT Code(s): ________________

    ICD-10-CM Code(s): ____________

39. Optic nerve decompression of the right eye.

    CPT Code(s): ________________

User to decide number of codes necessary to correctly answer the question.

Odd-numbered answers are located in Appendix B.

40. Removal of an embedded foreign body of the upper left eyelid.

    CPT Code: ________________

    ICD-10-CM Code: ____________

41. Myringoplasty of the left ear.

    CPT Code(s): ________________

42. Single-stage reconstruction of the right external auditory canal for congenital atresia.

    CPT Code: ________________

    ICD-10-CM Code: ____________

43. Left stapedectomy with footplate drill out.

    CPT Code(s): ________________

44. Excision of a lacrimal sac, left eye.

    CPT Code(s): ________________

REPORTS

In Appendix A of this workbook you will find a section titled Reports, which contains original reports. Read the reports indicated below and supply the appropriate CPT and ICD-10-CM codes on the following lines:

45. Report 85

    CPT Code: ________________

    ICD-10-CM Code: ____________

46. Report 86

    CPT Code(s): ________________

47. Report 87

    CPT Code(s): ________________

48. Report 88

    CPT Code(s): ________________

User to decide number of codes necessary to correctly answer the question.

Odd-numbered answers are located in Appendix B.

CHAPTER 24

Radiology

http://evolve.elsevier.com/Buck/step

THEORY

Match the following terms to the correct definitions:

1. _____ Anterior (ventral)
2. _____ Posterior (dorsal)
3. _____ Superior
4. _____ Inferior
5. _____ Medial
6. _____ Lateral

a. Toward the midline of the body

b. Toward the head or the upper part of the body; also known as cephalad or cephalic

c. In front of

d. Away from the midline of the body (to the side)

e. In back of

f. Away from the head or the lower part of the body; also known as caudad or caudal

Match the following radiographic procedures to the correct structures imaged:

7. _____ Fluoroscopy
8. _____ Magnetic resonance imaging (MRI)
9. _____ Tomography
10. _____ Xeroradiography
11. _____ Barium
12. _____ Biometry

a. Radiographic contrast medium

b. Procedure for viewing the interior of the body using x-rays and projecting the image onto a television screen

c. Photoelectric process of radiographs

d. Application of a statistical method to a biological fact

e. Procedure that uses nonionizing radiation to view the body in a cross-sectional view

f. Procedure that allows viewing of a single plane of the body by blurring out all but that particular level

Odd-numbered answers are located in Appendix B.

Match the following radiographic procedures to the correct structures imaged:

13. _____ Arthrography
14. _____ Cholangiography
15. _____ Cystography
16. _____ Discography
17. _____ Epididymography
18. _____ Hysterosalpingography
19. _____ Lymphangiography
20. _____ Myelography
21. _____ Urography
22. _____ Venography

a. Uterine cavity and fallopian tubes
b. Intervertebral joint
c. Kidneys, renal pelvis, ureters, and bladder
d. Bile ducts
e. Joint
f. Veins and tributaries
g. Subarachnoid space of the spine
h. Epididymis
i. Urinary bladder
j. Lymphatic vessels and nodes

PRACTICAL

Using the CPT and ICD-10-CM manuals, answer the following:

23. What is the unlisted diagnostic nuclear medicine code reported for cardiovascular procedures?

    CPT Code: ________________

24. What is the add-on code for the coronary artery transcatheter placement during coronary intravascular brachytherapy for delivery of the radiation device?

    Code: ________________

25. The modifier to indicate only the professional component was provided.

    Modifier: __________

26. The modifier to indicate only the technical component was provided.

    Modifier: __________

27. Supervision and interpretation of angiography, spinal artery, selective. Report radiology service only.

    CPT Code: ________________

Odd-numbered answers are located in Appendix B.

28. Radiological examination of the eye for foreign body.

    CPT Code: ________________

29. Radiological examination of mastoids, four views per side.

    CPT Code: ________________

30. Radiological examination of the ribs, unilateral, two views.

    CPT Code: ________________

31. MRI of the neck, with contrast material.

    CPT Code: ________________

32. Computed tomography of the thoracic spine, without contrast.

    CPT Code: ________________

33. Hip x-ray study, unilateral, two views.

    CPT Code: ________________

34. Complete four-view radiological examination of the wrist.

    CPT Code: ________________

35. Radiological examination of a surgical specimen.

    CPT Code: ________________

36. An established patient is seen in the clinic office complaining of severe headaches. To diagnose and treat the patient, the physician needs to identify a cause for these headaches. He performs a history and examination, low MDM, and orders a CT scan of the head. The clinic radiologist performed the x-ray in which contrast was used.

    CPT Codes: ________________ (physician), ________________ (radiologist)

37. A new patient is admitted to the hospital on an observation status after a fall at home. After talking to the patient and relatives and performing the examination, the physician finds that the patient has a number of symptoms that are usually due to an increase in intracranial pressure. The physician considers this patient's problems to be of moderately severe complexity. The MDM complexity is moderate. A CT scan of the brain without contrast is done. Brain lesions are discovered, and the physician advises radiation therapy. The patient is sent to the clinic's radiology department, where an A-scan bilateral ophthalmic biometry by ultrasound is done. The patient later has therapeutic radiology

Odd-numbered answers are located in Appendix B.

treatment planning that is simple. Later the patient has radiation treatment delivery to a single area up to 5 MeV. The patient continues with weekly radiology therapy management, five treatments.

CPT Codes: ____________, ____________,

____________, ____________, ____________,

____

38. A new patient is seen in the clinic for an office consult. The patient has a mass in the neck with related pain and dysphagia. The consulting physician performs an expanded problem-focused history and examination, and low-complexity decision making. A CT scan of the patient's neck is ordered. This was done with and without contrast.

    CPT Code(s): ____________

39. A patient was admitted to the hospital for removal of a pericardial clot. The physician orders a real-time chest ultrasound. Chest magnetic resonance (proton) imaging is also ordered (without contrast). A pericardiotomy is performed for removal of clot.

    CPT Code(s): ____________

40. Radiological examination, ankle, two views.

    CPT Code(s): ____________

41. X-ray of a 6-month-old's upper arm, two views.

    CPT Code(s): ____________

42. Unilateral selective pulmonary angiography, supervision and interpretation. Report radiology service only.

    CPT Code(s): ____________

43. Fluoroscopic guidance for needle placement.

    CPT Code(s): ____________

44. Computed tomography guidance for stereotactic localization.

    CPT Code(s): ____________

45. Transrectal ultrasound.

    CPT Code(s): ____________

User to decide number of codes necessary to correctly answer the question.

Odd-numbered answers are located in Appendix B.

46. Four-view x-ray of the lumbosacral spine.

CPT Code(s): ___________________

47. Myelography, cervical, radiological supervision and interpretation.

CPT Code(s): ___________________

48. Bilateral screening mammography.

CPT Code(s): ___________________

49. X-ray of the facial bones, two views.

CPT Code(s): ___________________

50. TMJ x-ray with mouth open and closed on one side of the mouth.

CPT Code(s): ___________________

51. X-ray of abdomen, two views.

CPT Code(s): ___________________

52. Placement of a long gastrointestinal tube, including fluoroscopy, radiological supervision, and interpretation. Report radiology service only.

CPT Code(s): ___________________

53. Venography, superior sagittal sinus, radiological supervision and interpretation for thrombosis of intracranial venous sinus. Report radiology service only.

CPT Code: ___________________

ICD-10-CM Code: _______________

54. Magnetic resonance spectroscopy for temporal meningioma, benign.

CPT Code: ___________________

ICD-10-CM Code: _______________

55. Endoluminal imaging of a noncoronary vessel, radiological supervision and interpretation due to renal artery stenosis.

CPT Code: ___________________

ICD-10-CM Code: _______________

User to decide number of codes necessary to correctly answer the question.

Odd-numbered answers are located in Appendix B.

56. Venography of unilateral extremity; radiological supervision and interpretation in a patient with end-stage renal disease on hemodialysis. Report radiology service only.

    CPT Code: ____________________

    ICD-10-CM Codes: ________________, ________________

REPORTS

In Appendix A of this workbook you will find a section titled Reports, which contains original reports. Read the reports indicated below and supply the appropriate CPT and ICD-10-CM codes on the following lines:

57. Report 45

    CPT Code: ____________________

    ICD-10-CM Code: ________________

58. Report 46

    CPT Code: ____________________

    ICD-10-CM Code: ________________

59. Report 47

    CPT Code: ____________________

    ICD-10-CM Code: ________________

60. Report 48

    CPT Code: ____________________

    ICD-10-CM Code: ________________

61. Report 49

    CPT Code(s): ____________________

    ICD-10-CM Code(s): ________________

62. Report 50

    CPT Code(s): ____________________

    ICD-10-CM Code(s): ________________

User to decide number of codes necessary to correctly answer the question.

Odd-numbered answers are located in Appendix B.

63. Report 51

CPT Code(s): ____________________

ICD-10-CM Code(s): ________________

64. Report 52

CPT Code(s): ____________________

ICD-10-CM Code(s): ________________

65. Report 53

CPT Code(s): ____________________

ICD-10-CM Code(s): ________________

User to decide number of codes necessary to correctly answer the question.

Odd-numbered answers are located in Appendix B.

CHAPTER 25

Pathology/Laboratory

http://evolve.elsevier.com/Buck/step

THEORY

Without the use of reference materials, answer the following:

1. In what section of the CPT manual will you find the codes to indicate the service of venipuncture? ________________

2. When a laboratory drug test is qualitative, it measures the ________________ of the drug.

3. When a laboratory drug test is quantitative, it measures the ________________ and the ________________ of a specific drug.

4. When coding an evocative/suppression test, you may have an E/M code to indicate a prolonged period of time the physician spends with the patient during the testing process or a report of the injection or infusion service. What other service may you need to report?

   ____

5. A sample of tissue from a suspect area that is examined by a pathologist is a specimen, a block is a frozen piece of the specimen, and a(n) ________________ is a slice of the frozen block.

6. How many levels of surgical pathology are there? __________

7. If one breast specimen is received for pathological analysis and the pathologist examines two blocks of the specimen, how many codes would be used to report the service of analysis? __________

Odd-numbered answers are located in Appendix B.

PRACTICAL

Using the CPT and ICD-10-CM manuals, code the following:

8. CARDIAC ENZYMES in a patient newly diagnosed with an acute inferior myocardial infarction.

Ref	*Range*	*Units*	*12/18/XX*
CPK	35-232 IU	69	0.0123
CKMB	0-10	ng/ml	1

CARDIAC MARKERS
12/18/XX +123 TROPONIN I <0.3 ng/ml

Troponin I Interpretation

≤0.4 ng/ml for apparently healthy individual

0.5-1.9 ng/ml for clinically diagnosed non-AMI patients

≥2.0 g/ml reasonably specific for AMI

CPT Codes: CPK, total: ________________

CKMB (creatine kinase, cardiac fraction):

____

Troponin, quantitative: ________________

ICD-10-CM Code: ______________

9. GENERAL BLOOD CHEMISTRY in a patient with dehydration, joint pains, and fever.

Ref	*Range*	*Units*	*10/30/XX 0620*	*10/27/XX 1855*
BUN	7-22	mg/dl		H 37
Sodium	136-145	mmol/L		138
Potassium	3.6-5.5	mmol/L		4.5
Creatinine	0.6-1.3	mg/dl	H 1.9	H 2.4
Uric acid	2.6-6.0	mg/dl	H 9.6	

CPT Codes: BUN: ________________

Sodium: ________________

Potassium: ________________

Creatinine: ________________

Uric acid: ________________

ICD-10-CM Codes: ______________, ______________, ______________

Odd-numbered answers are located in Appendix B.

10. An 84-year-old monitored for diagnoses of renal failure, anemia, and hypertension.

    CPT Codes: Labs include:

    Magnesium: ________________

    Iron: ________________

    Phosphorus: ________________

    Total protein serum: ________________

    ICD-10-CM Codes: ______________, ______________, ______________

11. A 48-year-old female patient with hyperlipidemia, currently on Lipitor.

    CPT Codes: Labs include:

    Hepatic function: ________________

    Lipid panel: ________________

    ICD-10-CM Code: ______________

12. A 20-year-old male in for labs due to chronic asthma.

    CPT Codes: Labs include:

    Theophylline: ________________

    ICD-10-CM Code: ______________

13. A 55-year-old male in for labs, total digoxin level for chronic atrial fibrillation.

    CPT Codes: Labs include:

    Digoxin; total: ________________

    ICD-10-CM Code:______________

REPORTS

In Appendix A of this workbook you will find a section titled Reports, which contains original reports. Read the reports indicated below and supply the appropriate CPT and ICD-10-CM codes on the following lines:

14. Report 54

    CPT Code(s): ________________

    ICD-10-CM Code(s): ______________

User to decide number of codes necessary to correctly answer the question.

Odd-numbered answers are located in Appendix B.

15. Report 55

    CPT Code(s): ________________

    ICD-10-CM Code(s): ______________

16. Report 56

    CPT Code(s): ________________

    ICD-10-CM Code(s): ______________

17. Report 57

    CPT Code(s): ________________

    ICD-10-CM Code(s): ______________

18. Report 58

    CPT Code(s): ________________

    ICD-10-CM Code(s): ______________

19. Report 59

    CPT Code(s): ________________

    ICD-10-CM Code(s): ______________

20. Report 60

    CPT Code(s): ________________

    ICD-10-CM Code(s): ______________

21. Report 61

    CPT Code(s): ________________

    ICD-10-CM Code(s): ______________

22. Report 62

    CPT Code(s): ________________

    ICD-10-CM Code(s): ______________

User to decide number of codes necessary to correctly answer the question.

Odd-numbered answers are located in Appendix B.

23. Report 63

    CPT Code(s): ____________________

    ICD-10-CM Code(s): ________________

24. Report 64

    CPT Code(s): ____________________

    ICD-10-CM Code(s): ________________

25. Report 65

    CPT Code(s): ____________________

    ICD-10-CM Code(s): ________________

26. Report 66

    CPT Code(s): ____________________

    ICD-10-CM Code(s): ________________

27. Report 67

    CPT Code(s): ____________________

    ICD-10-CM Code(s): ________________

User to decide number of codes necessary to correctly answer the question.

Odd-numbered answers are located in Appendix B.

CHAPTER 26

Medicine

http://evolve.elsevier.com/Buck/step

THEORY

Without the use of reference material, match the following terms to the correct definitions:

1. _____ Aphakia
2. _____ Echography
3. _____ Gonioscopy
4. _____ Hemodialysis
5. _____ Modality
6. _____ Nystagmus
7. _____ Optokinetic
8. _____ Percutaneous
9. _____ Phlebotomy
10. _____ Retrograde
11. _____ Subcutaneous
12. _____ Tonometry
13. _____ Transcutaneous
14. _____ Tympanometry

a. Entering by way of the skin
b. Moving backward or against the usual direction of flow
c. Through the skin
d. Cleansing of the blood outside the body
e. Procedure for evaluation of middle ear disorders
f. Rapid involuntary eye movements
g. Cutting into a vein
h. Use of a scope to examine the angles of the eye
i. Movement of the eye to objects moving in the visual field
j. Ultrasound procedure in which sound waves are bounced off an internal organ and the resulting image is recorded
k. Measurement of pressure or tension
l. Tissue below dermis, primarily fat cells that insulate the body
m. Absence of the lens of the eye
n. Treatment method

Odd-numbered answers are located in Appendix B.

Match the following administration methods for drugs:

15. _____ OTH	a. Subcutaneous
16. _____ IT	b. Inhalant solution
17. _____ IV	c. Various routes
18. _____ IM	d. Intrathecal
19. _____ SC	e. Intramuscular
20. _____ INH	f. Intravenous
21. _____ VAR	g. Other routes

Define the following terms:

22. Oscillating ____

23. Audiometry ____

24. Tympanometry ____

25. Electrocochleography ____

26. Orthoptic ____

27. Angioscopy ____

28. Electroretinography ____

29. Anomaloscope ____

30. Aphakia ____

31. Corneosclera ____

32. Cornea ____

33. Sclera ____

PRACTICAL

Using the CPT and ICD-10-CM manuals, code the following:

34. Three injections of allergen with the provision of the extract and professional service.

    CPT Code: ________________

Odd-numbered answers are located in Appendix B.

35. Two photo patch tests.

    CPT Code: __________________ × _______

36. Replacement of contact lenses.

    CPT Code: __________________

37. Patient is fitted for bifocal spectacles.

    CPT Code: __________________

38. Electrooculography with interpretation and report.

    CPT Code: __________________

39. Optokinetic nystagmus test.

    CPT Code: __________________

40. Positional nystagmus test, with recording, five positions.

    CPT Code: __________________

41. An esophagus acid reflux test with nasal catheter electrode placement for detection of gastroesophageal reflux.

    CPT Code: __________________

42. Peritoneal dialysis with two (repeated) physician evaluations.

    CPT Code: __________________

43. Hypnotherapy.

    CPT Code: __________________

44. Bernstein test for esophagitis.

    CPT Code: __________________

45. Evaluation of auditory rehabilitation status, 1 hour.

    CPT Code: __________________

46. A total of 50 minutes spent on family psychotherapy without the patient present.

    CPT Code: __________________

47. Hemodialysis access flow study to determine blood flow in grafts.

    CPT Code: __________________

Odd-numbered answers are located in Appendix B.

48. Puretone audiometry; air and bone.

    CPT Code: ________________

49. Insertion of a Swan-Ganz catheter.

    CPT Code: ________________

50. Electronic analysis for sick sinus syndrome of a single-chamber implantable defibrillator, with reprogramming (in person).

    CPT Code: ________________

    ICD-10-CM Code: ______________

51. Ventilation management for assist of breathing; second day for a hospital inpatient. The patient has a diagnosis of acute respiratory failure.

    CPT Code: ________________

    ICD-10-CM Code: ______________

52. Training for a prosthetic arm, 45 minutes.

    CPT Code(s): ________________

53. Conscious sedation provided by the same physician performing the diagnostic test on a 40-year-old patient for 30 minutes.

    CPT Code(s): ________________

54. GI tract intraluminal imaging from the esophagus through the ileum, with interpretation and report.

    CPT Code(s): ________________

55. Administration of two vaccines.

    CPT Code(s): ________________

56. The patient is being treated for bacterial endocarditis, on IV antibiotic therapy. The patient also has a new onset of ventricular flutter. The cardiologist documents a detailed history, detailed examination, and high medical decision making during this subsequent inpatient encounter.

    CPT Code(s): ________________

    ICD-10-CM Code(s): ______________

User to decide number of codes necessary to correctly answer the question.

Odd-numbered answers are located in Appendix B.

57. The service provided to the patient was an initial episode of care for an acquired atrial septal defect due to acute myocardial infarction of the inferolateral wall. The patient was admitted to the hospital for care.

    ICD-10-CM Codes: _______________, _______________

58. Arteriosclerosis of legs with intermittent claudication.

    ICD-10-CM Code: _______________

REPORTS

In Appendix A of this workbook you will find a section titled Reports, which contains original reports. Read the reports indicated below and supply the appropriate CPT and ICD-10-CM codes on the following lines:

59. Report 68

    CPT Code(s): ___________________

    ICD-10-CM Code(s): _______________

60. Report 69

    CPT Code(s): ___________________

    ICD-10-CM Code(s): _______________

61. Report 70

    CPT Code(s): ___________________

62. Report 71

    CPT Code(s): ___________________

63. Report 72

    CPT Code(s): ___________________

64. Report 73

    CPT Code(s): ___________________

65. Report 74

    CPT Code(s): ___________________

    ICD-10-CM Code(s): _______________

User to decide number of codes necessary to correctly answer the question.

Odd-numbered answers are located in Appendix B.

66. Report 75
    - CPT Code(s): ____________________

67. Report 76
    - CPT Code(s): ____________________
    - ICD-10-CM Code(s): ________________

68. Report 77
    - CPT Code(s): ____________________

69. Report 78
    - CPT Code(s): ____________________
    - ICD-10-CM Code(s): ________________

70. Report 79
    - CPT Code(s): ____________________
    - ICD-10-CM Code(s): ________________

71. Report 80
    - CPT Code(s): ____________________

72. Report 100
    - CPT Code(s): ____________________
    - ICD-10-CM Code(s): ________________

User to decide number of codes necessary to correctly answer the question.

Odd-numbered answers are located in Appendix B.

CHAPTER 27

Inpatient Coding

http://evolve.elsevier.com/Buck/step

THEORY

Without the use of reference material, complete the following:

1. In which setting would an ICD-10-PCS procedure code be assigned for a herniorrhaphy?

   Inpatient   Outpatient

2. In which setting would documentation in the discharge summary of a suspected condition be coded as if it exists?

   Inpatient   Outpatient

3. In which setting would a CPT code be assigned for a cataract extraction?

   Inpatient   Outpatient

4. A significant procedure must be performed in an operating room.

   True   False

5. The use of a POA indicator is optional.

   True   False

6. If a patient is admitted from outpatient surgery for a complication, the reason for the surgery is the principal diagnosis.

   True   False

7. When two or more diagnoses equally meet the definition for principal diagnosis, the one that the physician lists first should be assigned as the principal diagnosis.

   True   False

Odd-numbered answers are located in Appendix B.

8. A patient is admitted with syncope. The physician documents that the patient's syncope is due to orthostatic hypotension or bradycardia. Which diagnosis(es) should be reported?
   a. syncope
   b. syncope, orthostatic hypotension, bradycardia
   c. orthostatic hypotension, bradycardia
   d. bradycardia

9. Patient is admitted with right lower quadrant pain and anorexia due to acute appendicitis. Which diagnosis(es) should be reported?
   a. acute appendicitis
   b. right lower quadrant pain, appendicitis
   c. acute appendicitis, anorexia, right lower quadrant pain
   d. anorexia, acute appendicitis

10. If it is documented that the patient has a low magnesium level and magnesium supplements are ordered, the coder should:
    a. query the physician regarding the significance of the abnormal lab value and subsequent treatment
    b. add a code for abnormal lab value
    c. check with supervisor
    d. all of the above

Using Table 27-1 located in the main textbook, answer the following:

11. Altering the route of passage of the contents of a tubular body part is:
    a. alteration
    b. bypass
    c. change device in
    d. control postprocedural bleeding in

12. Cutting into a body part without draining fluids and/or gases from the body part in order to separate or transect a body part is:
    a. alteration
    b. detachment
    c. division
    d. change device in

13. Physical eradication of all or a portion of a body part by the direct use of energy, force, or a destructive agent is:
    a. division
    b. excision
    c. destruction
    d. resection

14. An example of fragmentation is:
    a. lithotripsy
    b. spinal fusion
    c. dermabrasion
    d. cutdown

Odd-numbered answers are located in Appendix B.

15. An example of an occlusion type of procedure is:
    a. clamping
    b. clipping
    c. ligation
    d. all of the above

SEQUENCING EXERCISES

Cases of Principal Diagnosis and Other Diagnoses

In the following cases, identify the principal diagnosis and other diagnoses using the ICD-10-CM Official Guidelines for Coding and Reporting. *This is a sequencing exercise, not a coding exercise. If there is only one diagnosis, write "none" for Other Diagnoses.*

16. Mr. Jones presents to the emergency department with complaints of leg pain, inflammation and swelling of the ankle and calf, and a fever. The day before he had been seen in the physician's office for treatment of cellulitis and was given antibiotics. Mr. Jones was admitted to the hospital for IV antibiotics.

    Principal Diagnosis: ___________________

    Other Diagnoses: ___________________

17. Mrs. Beatty was seen in her physician's office with a complaint of shortness of breath and chest pain. Dr. Adams admitted her with a diagnosis of congestive heart failure.

    Principal Diagnosis: ___________________

    Other Diagnoses: ___________________

18. Mr. Janes was admitted for colon resection for colon cancer and also had chemotherapy following surgery. Mr. Janes complained of joint pain while in the hospital, and an MRI showed metastases to bone.

    Principal Diagnosis: ___________________

    Other Diagnoses: ___________________

19. Mrs. Anderson had a hysterectomy and bilateral oophorectomy for ovarian cancer 1 week ago. It is planned that the patient will undergo chemotherapy. The patient is now admitted with internal hemorrhaging from the surgery site.

    Principal Diagnosis: ___________________

    Other Diagnoses: ___________________

Odd-numbered answers are located in Appendix B.

20. Miss Nelson is admitted for a D&C for menorrhagia. During her preoperative physical examination, the physician notices she has a fever and her lungs are congested. He cancels surgery because the patient shows symptoms of acute bronchitis.

    Principal Diagnosis: ____________________

    Other Diagnoses: ____________________

21. Jackie Jones was cooking at home and spilled a pot of boiling water on her arms, legs, and stomach. She presented to the emergency department with second-degree burns of the thighs and third-degree burns of the arms and stomach. She was admitted and taken directly to surgery.

    Principal Diagnosis: ____________________

    Other Diagnoses: ____________________

22. Mr. Anderson regularly sees a physician and is on medication for management of his chronic bronchitis. Last night he was complaining of coughing and difficulty breathing. He was admitted with a diagnosis of chronic bronchitis with acute exacerbation.

    Principal Diagnosis: ____________________

    Other Diagnoses: ____________________

23. Mrs. Smith is at 32 weeks' gestation and complaining of stomach cramps and diarrhea × 36 hours. She is admitted for rehydration with IV fluids and is diagnosed with dehydration and gastroenteritis. Pregnancy is thought to be incidental.

    Principal Diagnosis: ____________________

    Other Diagnoses: ____________________

PRINCIPAL DIAGNOSIS

Provide the principal diagnosis code, the procedure code, and any additional diagnosis codes for the following:

24. **HISTORY OF PRESENT ILLNESS:** The patient is a 52-year-old male who was involved in an interpersonal altercation at approximately 1:30 in the morning. He presented to the emergency department with complaints of pain and swelling to the right side of the face. The patient had been struck multiple times with the butt end of a handgun. He denied loss of consciousness. The attack was witnessed, and the witnesses also claimed there was no loss of consciousness. He presented with pain and swelling on the right side of his face in the temporal region and in the right eye region. He had a small abrasion on the top

Odd-numbered answers are located in Appendix B.

of his head and on the right forehead. No lacerations were noted. He had no diplopia. The past medical history and past surgical history were noncontributory. The patient was taking no medications and had no allergies.

HOSPITAL COURSE: Admission x-rays and CT scan revealed a nondisplaced right zygoma fracture and an orbital floor fracture with slight limitation on physical examination of his upward gaze. He was taken to the operating room for exploration and placement of a Silastic implant to the right orbital floor fracture, which was accomplished without difficulty and without complication. The patient tolerated the procedure well. Postoperative course was uncomplicated. He received IV antibiotics throughout his stay in the hospital.

FINAL DIAGNOSIS: Right orbital fracture; right zygoma fracture; abrasion of head.

ICD-10-CM PRINCIPAL DIAGNOSIS and CODE: ____________________

ICD-10-CM OTHER DIAGNOSES and CODES:

____________________, ____________________, ____________________,

____

ICD-10-PCS PROCEDURE CODE: ____________________

25. **HISTORY OF PRESENT ILLNESS:** The patient is a 69-year-old, right-handed male who presents with a 4-day history of severe right-sided headache, visual blurring, and diplopia. The patient was seen in the ENT clinic for discharge from his right ear of 2 days' duration, diagnosed to be otitis externa on the day of admission. The patient was subsequently transferred from the clinic to the emergency department. The patient denied a history of seizure, motor or sensory deficit, nausea or vomiting, trauma, or speech difficulties. Past medical history of sinusitis for many years. Current medications are none. Allergies, none.

    PHYSICAL EXAMINATION: HEENT: Right pupil 3 mm, nonreactive. Left pupil 2 mm, reactive. Disconjugate gaze present. Right ptosis. Oropharynx clear without lesions. The neck is supple without lymphadenopathy or thyromegaly. Heart: regular rate and rhythm without murmurs or gallops. Lungs clear to percussion and auscultation. The neurological examination: awake, alert, oriented times three, follows three simple commands. Cranial nerves, partial right third nerve palsy with ptosis, 3-mm nonreactive right pupil, right medial gaze with disconjugate extraocular eye movement. Motor is 5/5 throughout without drift. Finger test is within normal limits. The sensory is intact to fine touch and proprioception: cerebral examination within normal limits.

Odd-numbered answers are located in Appendix B.

HOSPITAL COURSE: Patient was admitted with suspicion of intracranial aneurysm. On the following day, the patient underwent a three-vessel cerebral angiogram that demonstrated a posterior communicating artery aneurysm and questionable anterior communicating artery aneurysm. The patient underwent a right craniotomy for clipping of right posterior communicating artery aneurysm and anterior communicating artery aneurysm. Postoperatively, the patient was observed in the surgical intensive care unit until his mental status was stabilized. The palsy and ptosis noted preoperatively resolved during the postsurgical course. The patient has been ambulating without assistance and tolerating food well. The patient was also seen by the ENT service during the hospitalization for his otitis externa, and their recommendations were followed.

FINAL DIAGNOSES: Right posterior communicating artery aneurysm; anterior communicating artery aneurysm; right otitis externa.

ICD-10-CM PRINCIPAL DIAGNOSIS and CODE: ____________________

ICD-10-CM OTHER DIAGNOSIS and CODE: ____________________

ICD-10-PCS PROCEDURE CODE: ____________________

Odd-numbered answers are located in Appendix B.

APPENDIX A

Reports

NOTE: These reports are meant to be referenced as exercises at the end of most *Workbook* chapters. Every report is assigned at least once, with odd-numbered question answers being provided in the corresponding *Workbook* chapter answer key.

1. EMERGENCY DEPARTMENT REPORT

The patient is a 32-year-old G-5, P-4, female at 36 weeks and 4 days by last menstrual period, who comes in to the emergency room complaining of a 4-day history of urinary frequency and urgency with cloudy urine. She is also complaining of some low back pain × 5 days. She denies burning, itching, pain with urination. She denies fever and chills. She has also had some nausea and vomiting over the same period. She last vomited yesterday. She vomited twice, she states, and, this past Friday, 4 days ago, twice. She has not vomited today. She has had good fluid intake. She has had a slightly decreased appetite, she states. The patient states that she has had some UTIs this pregnancy × 2. Otherwise, she has had an uncomplicated pregnancy.

The patient denies a history of hypertension, diabetes, and pre-eclampsia. She states she has had some irregular contractions, no real contractions today. She denies vaginal bleeding. She denies gush of fluid. She denies abdominal pain. She has had good fetal movement. She has not had headaches, visual changes, or abdominal pain.

PHYSICAL EXAMINATION: Blood pressure 119/66, temperature 36.5, pulse 86, respiratory rate 18. HEENT: Within normal limits. CHEST: Clear to auscultation bilaterally. HEART: Regular rate and rhythm without murmur, rub, or gallop. ABDOMEN: Gravida, nontender. Vertex. EXTREMITIES: The patient has 1+ pitting edema bilaterally to the knee. On cervical examination, the patient was 1-2 cm, long, –1 station. Fetal heart tones are 130's with accels. *(Average fetal heart rate is 120-160, so this is not an abnormal rate.)* No obvious contractions on the monitor. No flank tenderness to palpation.

LABORATORY DATA: Urinalysis is done and revealed yellow, turbid urine, specific gravity of 1.022, 100 protein, positive nitrite, moderate hemoglobin, large amount of leukocytes, 5-10 red cells, 3+ bacteria, too numerous to count white cells.

ASSESSMENT: This is a 32-year-old, G-5, P-4 at 36 and 4/5 weeks, with a urinary tract infection. The patient was given a prescription for Macrobid 100 mg p.o. b.i.d. × 7 days. She is instructed to follow up with her OB doctor in 2 days for recheck of her urine and her symptomatology. She was given labor precautions. She was advised that, if she develops fevers, back pain, worsening symptomatology, she should come in immediately for evaluation.

2. DISCHARGE SUMMARY

DIAGNOSES include:

1. Chronic pelvic pain secondary to pelvic metastatic clear cell carcinoma of unknown primary location.
2. Vena cava syndrome post placement of Hickman catheter.
3. Anemia due to chronic disease.
4. Hypertension.

HOSPITAL COURSE: The patient is a 78-year-old female whom we have been following in our clinic for hypertension and also chronic pudendal nerve pain. She had been recently diagnosed with pelvic metastatic clear cell carcinoma, which her primary location is unknown at this time. She will be discussing this further after the pathology reports are read. During her hospital stay a Hickman catheter was placed in order to have IV access for pain medication or future cancer therapy. She was also admitted for chronic pain. She did develop swelling of her arms and neck. She was brought to interventional radiology, and she did have venography, and the Hickman catheter was removed. Her swelling to her arms and neck have decreased greatly. She denies any shortness of breath. No choking sensation as previously noted. Her pain has been managed well with fentanyl patch at 175 mcg. She has also been on IV heparin therapy for anticoagulation following the vena cava syndrome. Today, the patient has been having complaints of nausea. She did get some dexamethasone IV for her nausea, which did improve later this morning. Her blood pressure has been under good control. Her labs today include a WBC of 5.18, hemoglobin 7.8, hematocrit 23.7, protime 14.4, INR 1.5, PTT 39.6, BUN 6, sodium 139, potassium 4.2, CO_2 27.2.

DISCHARGE PLANS:

1. IV heparin is discontinued. She will be switched over to Lovenox 1 mg/kg subcutaneously daily. The patient will have Home Health to help her set up these injections.
2. She will continue with the fentanyl patch 175 mcg for the pain.
3. She will receive 40,000 units subcutaneously of Procrit at the Cancer Center one time per week. We will follow up in 3 days with a CBC and a basic metabolic panel.
4. Follow-up appointment at the Hypertension Center on November 2 at 10:30 in the morning. Will also check CBC and a basic metabolic panel, PTT, PT, and INR before that appointment.
5. Hold potassium supplements for now.
6. She may use Phenergan p.o. 12.5 mg 1-2 tablets p.o. p.r.n. every 6 hours for nausea.

7. She does have a follow-up appointment set up with Dr. Smith on Friday, 10/29/XX, to discuss her pathology results and decide what further treatment is to be done. He will also be discussing plans with Dr. Sticca.

The above plan was discussed with the patient and her husband. They seem to be in agreement. They were encouraged to call our office with any questions or concerns.

DISCHARGE MEDICATIONS:

1. Will continue home medications.
2. Phenergan 12.5 1-2 tabs p.o. p.r.n. every 6 hours for nausea.
3. Lovenox 1 mg/kg subcutaneously every 24 hours. *(treatment for thrombosis—blood clots)*
4. Fentanyl patch 175 mcg to be changed every 3 days. *(analgesic)*
5. Epogen 40,000 units subcutaneously weekly at the Cancer Center. *(treatment for anemia)*

Total time spent with the patient today is 60 minutes.

3. CLINIC CHART NOTE

HISTORY: This 16-year-old female is seen today after falling off a curb and twisting her right ankle. She is normally a patient of Dr. Anderson, who is out of town this week. *(Both physicians are of the same specialty and in the same clinic.)* She states that she has pain surrounding the entire foot and ankle. Seems unable or unwilling to bear weight.

PHYSICAL EXAMINATION: Ankle and foot examined. Foot is warm to touch. Some swelling and bruising noted around the lateral aspect of the ankle. X-ray is negative for fracture.

IMPRESSION: Sprained right ankle. (MDM complexity straightforward)

PLAN: Elevation; ice to affected area. Weight bearing only as tolerated. Return for follow-up p.r.n.

4. ADMIT INPATIENT

This is a 19-year-old with a living-related donor kidney transplant as of last month and admitted to hospital for possible sepsis.

HISTORY: This patient has type 1 diabetes and had been on dialysis for a number of years before transplantation. She received her mother's kidney on the 14th of last month from the Medical Center Transplant Program in Dallas. She was there this Tuesday for a transplant visit and apparently did not feel well, but they were not certain whether this was a problem or not; but they did go ahead and do blood cultures and called the public health nurse, who was visiting the patient today, and said that one of the cultures was positive for group B strep. The home health nurse called me and stated that the patient has really gone downhill the past few days and was quite fatigued with generalized malaise. Denied cough, fever, or shaking chills but looked poor overall, and the nurse was quite concerned. We recommended she be brought here for evaluation and treatment as an emergency. After arrival here, she was in no acute distress. Initially, she had bibasilar crackles on deep breathing; however, most of these cleared. I cannot hear any significant pulmonary abnormality on auscultation or percussion. Her heart is normal regular rhythm. No significant murmurs, rubs, S3, or S4. Her abdomen is negative. Her left lower-quadrant kidney is nontender. She has no edema and no lateralizing neural sounds. She is a little lethargic. She does not feel warm. Apparently she is afebrile. Her blood pressure is normal, and she is not tachycardic, but she simply does not look well. Past history, social history, and system review are per our recent old chart and noncontributory at present.

MEDICATIONS: See med sheet.

CLINICAL IMPRESSION: One positive group B strep blood culture, significance, and/or etiology to be determined. My impression at this time is probably a significant finding, and I suspect that this will become a progressive syndrome if not treated.

ADDITIONAL DIAGNOSES:

1. Living-related donor kidney transplant.
2. Diabetes mellitus type 1.
3. Hypertension.

PLAN: Repeat culture. Culture urine. Do chest x-ray stat and repeat lab. Will empirically treat pending results at this time.

5. NEPHROLOGY HOSPITAL PROGRESS NOTE

This patient continues to be stable with no new problems. Her cultures remain negative, and she remains afebrile. Her clearance is pending, but she certainly has settled down nicely. The main problem we are having is with her diabetic management. It simply is not working with the former twice a day of 70/30 insulin plus a nighttime Lantus. I think we should go one way or the other, and we will go to Humalog before each meal, starting with an estimated dose of 15 per meal and 40 of Lantus in the evening, and we will titrate from there. We will get Accu-Cheks before each meal to reflect the previous meal's dose of Humalog and adjust it accordingly. Other than that, tomorrow we will review her case with infectious disease with regard to the duration of her antibiotic therapy. Thus far, our cultures have remained negative; however, the positive group B strep is not the type of typical contaminant you get in a blood culture, and we must take it at face value.

Time spent re-evaluating the patient, reviewing the chart, and rearranging diabetic management was 25 minutes; more than half of the time was coordination.

6. OPERATIVE REPORT

PREOPERATIVE DIAGNOSIS: Scar right parietal region.

POSTOPERATIVE DIAGNOSIS: Same.

SURGICAL FINDINGS: 3 × 1 cm elevated scar right parietal region of scalp.

SURGICAL PROCEDURE: Excision scar of scalp.

SURGEON: Dr. Harold Wallingford

ANESTHESIA: General endotracheal anesthesia, plus 2 cc of 1% Xylocaine and 1:100,000 epinephrine.

PROCEDURE: The scalp was prepped with Betadine scrub and solution, draped in the routine sterile fashion. The lesion was anesthetized with 2 cc of 1% Xylocaine with 1:100,000 epinephrine, mostly for the epinephrine effect. After a wait of 4 minutes the lesion was excised, bleeding was electrocoagulated, the wound was closed with vertical mattress sutures of 3-0 Prolene. Surgicel and antibiotic ointment were applied. The patient tolerated the procedure well and left the operating room in good condition.

PATHOLOGY REPORT LATER INDICATED: Benign tissue.

7. OPERATIVE REPORT

PREOPERATIVE DIAGNOSIS: Lipoma left posterior axillary fold.

POSTOPERATIVE DIAGNOSIS: Same.

SURGICAL FINDINGS: 6 cm diameter lipoma attached to latissimus dorsi muscle.

PROCEDURE PERFORMED: Excision of lipoma left posterior axillary fold.

ANESTHESIA: General endotracheal anesthesia with 5 cc 1% Xylocaine with 1:100,000 epinephrine injected along the incision line.

COMPLICATIONS: None.

SPONGE AND NEEDLE COUNT: Correct.

DRAINS: One #10 Jackson-Pratt.

DESCRIPTION OF PROCEDURE: The patient's posterior arm was prepped with Betadine scrub and solution and draped in the routine sterile fashion. About 5 cc of 1% Xylocaine with 1:100,000 epinephrine were injected along the incision line. Dissection was carried down to the site of the lipomatous mass, which was dissected free of the skin and dissected free of the muscle using sharp dissection with very little bleeding. Bleeding was electrocoagulated. Because of the size of the pocket, we inserted a drain and brought it out through a separate stab wound incision using a #10 Jackson-Pratt drain. The wound was then closed, effectively closing the dead space with interrupted 2-0 Monocryl, subcuticular 3-0 Monocryl, and a few twists of 4-0 Prolene. Dressing consisted of Kerlix fluffs, Elastoplast, a clavicle strap, and a sling. The patient tolerated the procedure well and left the area in good condition.

PATHOLOGY REPORT LATER INDICATED: See Report 60.

8. OPERATIVE REPORT

PREOPERATIVE DIAGNOSIS: Pyogenic granuloma, sinus tract, buttock.

POSTOPERATIVE DIAGNOSIS: Multiple sinus tracts, one extending inferiorly about 7 × 3 cm in diameter, one extending to the right approximately 4 × 3 cm, and one 4 × 3 cm extending to the left of 4 × 3 cm.

SURGICAL FINDINGS: As above, plus (benign) granulation tissue present in a capsule of multiple sinus tracts. Sinus tracts measured a total of about 15 × 8 cm in their total dimensions.

SURGICAL PROCEDURE: Partial unroofing of sinus tracts. *(This is a full-thickness debridement.)*

ANESTHESIA: General endotracheal.

DESCRIPTION OF PROCEDURE: The patient was intubated and turned in the prone position. A probe was inserted in the sinus cavity, and dissection was carried down to this. I encountered a piece of chronically infected granulation tissue coming out of a hole, in which I stuck the probe, but this continued for a distance longer than the probe and accordingly, I put my finger in this, and this extended down the length of my index finger *(i.e., about 7-8 cm by about 3 cm in width).* I left this intact, because this would necessitate extensive dissection of 15 sq cm of subcutaneous tissue, and we have no blood on this patient at this time. We then unroofed two other sinus cavities, and packed this opened with 2-inch vaginal packing and applied a dressing and Kerlix plus an Elastoplast. Estimated blood loss: 25 cc. The patient seemed to tolerate the procedure well and left the operating room in good condition.

Coder's Query: It is unclear from the documentation exactly what the procedure was that the physician performed. The coder queried the physician and asked for additional information to ensure correct coding. The physician explained that the patient has a recurrent history of pyogenic granuloma of the buttock with sinus tracts that have, as in this instance, required a subcutaneous tissue debridement.

9. OPERATIVE REPORT

PREOPERATIVE DIAGNOSIS: Mass, right breast.

POSTOPERATIVE DIAGNOSIS: Mass, right breast.

OPERATIVE PROCEDURE: Right breast mass excision.

PROCEDURE: With the female patient under general anesthesia, the breast and chest were prepped and draped in a sterile manner. An elliptical incision was made in the central portion of the breast about the palpated mass, including the area of the nipple. This was excised all the way down to the fascia of the breast and then submitted for frozen section. Frozen section revealed a carcinoma of the breast with what appeared to be a good margin all the way around it. We then maintained hemostasis with electrocautery and proceeded to close the breast tissue using 2-0 and 3-0 chromic. The skin was closed using 4-0 Vicryl in a subcuticular manner. Steri-Strips were applied. The patient tolerated the procedure well and was discharged from the operating room in stable condition.

PATHOLOGY REPORT LATER INDICATED: Primary, malignant neoplasm.

10. OPERATIVE REPORT

PREOPERATIVE DIAGNOSIS: Neck injury, closed posterior cord syndrome caused by a fracture due to a motor vehicle accident.

POSTOPERATIVE DIAGNOSIS: Same as preoperative.

PROCEDURE PERFORMED: Placement of halo crown and vest.

ANESTHESIA: Local.

SURGICAL INDICATIONS: This 56-year-old patient was in a motor vehicle accident, hitting a tree. He was the driver and appears to have sustained a cervical spinal cord fracture at C1–4. He could not be placed in a neck collar because he has a short, thick neck and also because he had a tracheostomy tube. The patient would not be stabilized with traction as he has a distraction injury. It was indicated to place him in a halo vest and crown to immobilize his neck.

PROCEDURE: The hair was shaved behind both ears. There was a sterile prep done along the forehead region and the region behind both ears. The halo crown was then positioned and stabilized with the three positioners anteriorly and two laterally. I then injected Xylocaine behind both ears and along the supraorbital ridge laterally. I then placed the four pins and torqued them to 8 pounds per sq inch. The hexagonal lock nuts were then tightened. The patient tolerated this well without any apparent complications. The halo vest was then connected to the crown. The crown was placed. A large vest was used but this was still too small for the patient, and on the right side the vest had to be tied with string until some permanent straps could be fashioned by orthotics. During the placement of the vest, I maintained the neck in neutral position, and at no time was there any rotation or flexion or extension of the neck.

11. OPERATIVE REPORT

PREOPERATIVE DIAGNOSIS: Bulky free flap, right heel.

POSTOPERATIVE DIAGNOSIS: Same.

SURGICAL FINDINGS: 10.5×8.5 cm area of redundant fat of flap of right heel.

PROCEDURE PERFORMED: Defatting of flap of right heel with excision of redundant skin (benign).

ANESTHESIA: General endotracheal anesthesia.

POSITION: Prone.

ESTIMATED BLOOD LOSS: Negligible.

DESCRIPTION OF PROCEDURE: The patient was intubated and turned into prone position. The right foot and lower leg were prepped with Betadine scrub and solution and were draped in the routine sterile fashion. The medial aspect of the flap was elevated excising the old scar in the process, and the flap was elevated to about 60% of its extent to include all of the redundant fat that was within the flap. We removed about 1.5 cm thickness of flap from the bottom of the flap and left a layer of padding of about a centimeter on the bed. Hemostasis was secured, and then we closed the wound with a combination of plain 3-0 Prolene and horizontal mattress sutures and some horizontal half mattress sutures of 3-0 Prolene. We dressed the wound temporarily with Kerlix and Kling. Dr. Miller will then proceed with his portion of the procedure.

12. OPERATIVE REPORT

PREOPERATIVE DIAGNOSIS: Ischial pressure ulcer with massive ischioperineal and buttock sinus.

POSTOPERATIVE DIAGNOSIS: Same.

FINDINGS: There was a 2 cm open surgical ulcer extending down and connecting with an 8 × 30 cm diameter granulation-lined sinus cavity.

SURGICAL PROCEDURE: Excision of left ischial ulcer with total excision of 8 × 30 cm sinus of the buttock, perineal, and ischial areas.

ANESTHESIA: General endotracheal.

ESTIMATED BLOOD LOSS: 400 ml.

FLUIDS: 2 liters Ringer's lactate.

DRAINS: None.

COMPLICATION: None.

SPONGE AND NEEDLE COUNTS: Correct.

DESCRIPTION: The patient was intubated and turned in the right lateral decubitus position. I injected about 10 ml of 1% Xylocaine with 1:100,000 epinephrine around the surface ulcer and made incisions down to the granulation tissue, keeping this intact. I opened the skin over the extent of the sinus tracts proximally and distally, trying to keep this in line with a potential Y-V advancement flap, and with some difficulty and remarkable bleeding around what appeared to be the sacrum, I was able to remove virtually intact the entire ulcer, covered with chronically infected granulation tissue. This granulation tissue was poor quality and had an unhealthy appearance. A piece of this was dropped in a culture tube as was a piece of what appeared to be the sacrum, which was quite sclerotic and consistent with an osteomyelitis of the sacrum. Following this extensive removal of the ulcer, I cauterized all of the bleeding and did a stick-tie on one of the bleeders with 2-0 Vicryl. I then sprayed the base with topical thrombin, packed the wound open with 2-inch vaginal packing soaked in 5/10th percent metronidazole, and then put several #2 Prolene sutures to keep the packing in place and to help seal off the wound from the fecal contamination. I put a Vi-Drape over this and then dressed it with Kerlix fluffs, ABD pads, and Elastoplast. The patient tolerated the procedure well and left the area in good condition.

PATHOLOGY REPORT LATER INDICATED: See Report 62.

13. OPERATIVE REPORT

PROCEDURE: Steroid injection.

INDICATIONS: Left shoulder bursitis, rotator cuff syndrome.

PROCEDURE: This procedure was done in the procedure area in the outpatient department of the hospital. After obtaining consent, area of the left shoulder was prepped in the usual fashion with Betadine. 6 cc of 1% lidocaine with 1 cc of Kenalog was injected in the left subacromial bursa without difficulty. The patient tolerated the procedure well without immediate complications. There was moderate relief of pain afterward. The patient was advised to call me if she gets any signs of infection, such as fever, chills, erythema, or swelling. She will call me in 3 days and tell me how she is doing.

14. OPERATIVE REPORT

PREOPERATIVE DIAGNOSIS: Deltoid muscle pain and swelling.

POSTOPERATIVE DIAGNOSIS: Same.

PRELIMINARY NOTE: This patient was brought down to the operating room on the ventilator, and we used the operating room because of this.

OPERATIVE NOTE: With the patient in the supine position we prepped and draped the left deltoid region. After infiltration with 0.5% Marcaine with epinephrine, a vertical incision was made over the palpated muscular belly. Sharp dissection was carried down to the muscle belly and then we freed up a segment of muscle. We did infiltrate the ends of the muscle away from where we were taking our biopsy with the Marcaine. A segment of muscle was then isolated between clamps and then we excised the segment of muscle and submitted it immediately to the histology department for proper processing. The ends of the muscle were ligated using 2-0 chromic and then the muscular fascia was brought together using 2-0 chromic. Subcutaneous tissue was closed using 2-0 chromic and then the skin was closed using 4-0 nylon in running mattress fashion. A sterile dressing was applied. The patient tolerated the procedure well and was discharged from the operating room in stable condition. At the end of the procedure all sponges and instruments were accounted for.

PATHOLOGY REPORT LATER INDICATED: See Report 59.

15. OPERATIVE REPORT

PREOPERATIVE DIAGNOSIS: Left distal radius fracture.

POSTOPERATIVE DIAGNOSIS: Same.

PROCEDURE PERFORMED: Closed reduction and pinning of closed left distal radius fracture.

COMPLICATIONS: None.

INDICATIONS: This is a 31-year-old female who fell yesterday down a flight of stairs, fracturing her left wrist. She has been stabilized in the intensive care unit throughout the day today. Her injuries include a comminuted intra-articular left distal radius fracture, displaced.

The patient's x-rays are consistent with a displaced comminuted intra-articular distal radius fracture. This is an unstable fracture and requires reduction and probable pinning versus open reduction and internal fixation.

Prior to the procedure, I spoke with the patient regarding her left wrist. We discussed management options in detail, and I recommended proceeding with a closed reduction versus pinning versus ORIF of her left distal radius. The procedure, alternatives, risks, benefits, and expected rehab course were discussed in detail. She understood the implications of surgery and wished to proceed.

PROCEDURE: The patient was brought to the operating room and placed supine on the operating room table. She underwent general anesthesia. The left wrist was initially examined under fluoroscopic guidance. There was comminution and intra-articular involvement. There was dorsal tilt of 30 degrees, shortening, and angulation. We performed a closed reduction with longitudinal traction, manipulation at the fracture, and volar flexion. We obtained a near anatomic reduction with maintenance of radial length and inclination. Additionally, there was neutral tilt. However, with release of traction, there was some instability to the fracture with some residual collapse. Subsequently, the left upper extremity was prepped and draped in standard surgical fashion. Under fluoroscopic guidance, a closed reduction was again obtained. Two separate 0.062 K-wires were placed through the radial styloid, across the main fracture, and into the more proximal shaft. Both of these screws had good fixation in the bone.

Final fluoroscopic views were obtained confirming a near anatomic reduction. The pins were then cut off 1 cm above skin level. The pin sites were dressed with Xeroform gauze and adequately padded. The left upper extremity was then placed into a well-padded and molded long-arm cast with the wrist in neutral, forearm neutral, and elbow 90 degrees.

The patient was awakened from anesthesia and tolerated the procedure well. She was transferred back to the recovery room in stable condition. There were no intraoperative complications for the wrist portion of the procedure.

16. OPERATIVE REPORT

PREOPERATIVE DIAGNOSIS: Degenerative joint disease, medial compartment plus old meniscal tear.

POSTOPERATIVE DIAGNOSIS: Posterior horn tear, old, medial meniscus; diffuse grade 3-4 chondromalacia, medial femoral condyle 0-90 degrees; and grade 4 chondromalacia, superior half of the patella.

PROCEDURE PERFORMED: Arthroscopy and partial arthroscopic meniscectomy, right knee.

OPERATIVE PROCEDURE: After suitable general anesthesia had been achieved, the patient's right knee was prepped and draped in the usual manner. Before prepping, a thigh tourniquet was applied; after draping, it was inflated to 300 mm Hg. No inflow cannula was used. Arthroscope was inserted through an anteromedial portal. The lateral compartment was examined. Everything looked good. Examination of the notch revealed some inflated synovial tissue, which was cauterized with a radiofrequency probe. Examination of the medial compartment revealed a horizontal cleavage tear and flap tear of the posterior horn of the medial meniscus. Using a combination of punch and shaver, the unstable meniscus was excised and contoured. The tibial surfaces revealed a small area of water by the anterior horn of the meniscus. Femoral surfaces showed diffuse wear of grade 3 with occasional areas of grade 4 chondromalacia from 0 to 90 degrees. Examination of the patellofemoral joint revealed very good looking articular surfaces on the inferior half of the patella in the trochlea. However, there was essentially bare bone on the superior half of the articular surface.

The knee joint was then thoroughly irrigated, and the arthroscope removed. Stab wounds were closed with 3-0 nylon. A dressing was then applied. Tourniquet was released, after which good circulation was noted to return to the foot. The patient tolerated the procedure well and returned to the recovery room in stable condition.

PATHOLOGY REPORT LATER INDICATED: Benign meniscus tissue and bone chips.

17. OPERATIVE REPORT

PREOPERATIVE DIAGNOSIS: Subtrochanteric fracture, closed, right hip.

POSTOPERATIVE DIAGNOSIS: Subtrochanteric fracture, right hip.

PROCEDURE PERFORMED: Open reduction internal fixation of subtrochanteric fracture, right hip.

ANESTHESIA: Spinal.

FINDINGS: The patient had a displaced comminuted subtrochanteric fracture of her right hip. We were able to align this fairly well and hold this in place with a dynamic hip screw device.

PROCEDURE: While under spinal anesthetic, the patient was placed in the supine position on the fracture table, where gentle traction was applied to the right leg and the left leg was abducted. We visualized the fracture using the C-arm image intensifier. We were satisfied with the position and then prepped the patient's right hip with Betadine and draped it in a sterile fashion. She was given 1 g of Kefzol intravenously preoperatively.

We then created a longitudinal incision over the lateral aspect of the right hip and carried the dissection down through the subcutaneous tissue. The fascia was incised longitudinally, and we reflected the vastus lateralis anteriorly, exposing the lateral aspect of the femoral shaft. We were able to palpate the fracture and found that it was significantly displaced. We attempted to reduce this. We then drilled a 9/64-inch hole in the lateral aspect of the femoral shaft through which we advanced a guide pin into the femoral head at an angle of 135 degrees to the femoral shaft. We then passed a reamer over this and reamed to a depth of 110 mm and inserted a 100-mg lag screw into the femoral head. We attempted to position this lag screw in the center of the femoral head as best as possible as seen in both the AP and lateral views.

We then attached a 135-degree four-hole side plate and secured this plate to the femoral shaft using four cortical screws. We then released the traction of the leg and inserted a compressing screw into the end of the lag screw. The resultant fixation appeared to be quite satisfactory. We again used the C-arm image intensifier to evaluate the fracture and found it to be very acceptable.

We then thoroughly irrigated the area with saline and placed a Hemovac drain deep to the fascia. We then closed the fascia using 0 Vicryl and the subcutaneous tissue with 2-0 Vicryl. The skin was closed using skin staples. A sterile Xeroform dressing was applied, and the patient was then taken from the operating room in good condition breathing spontaneously. The final sponge and needle counts were correct. She will be continued on IV Kefzol for at least 24 hours.

18. OPERATIVE REPORT

PREOPERATIVE DIAGNOSIS: Comminuted fracture, right olecranon process of the ulna.

POSTOPERATIVE DIAGNOSIS: Comminuted fracture, right olecranon process of the ulna.

PROCEDURE PERFORMED: Open reduction internal fixation, right olecranon fracture.

ANESTHESIA: General.

FINDINGS: The patient had a markedly comminuted displaced fracture of his right olecranon. He had involved a significant portion of the articular surface. We were able to reassemble the major fragments; however, we did have to debride some of the articular cartilage from the joint, which resulted in a defect in the articular cartilage of some significance.

PROCEDURE: While under a general anesthetic, the patient was placed in the supine position on the operating room table, where his right arm was prepped with Betadine and draped in a sterile fashion. We used an Esmarch bandage to exsanguinate the arm, and a tourniquet on the limb was inflated to 250 mm Hg. The total tourniquet time ended up being 43 minutes.

We created a longitudinal incision over the posterior aspect of the elbow, skirting to the radial side of the olecranon. We carried the dissection down through the subcutaneous tissue and easily identified the fracture site as the periosteum was torn over this area. We used suction to irrigate the hematoma. Several pieces of articular cartilage lay in the joint, which we debrided, and there was some other cancellous bone, which we debrided as well because it was lying loose in the joint. We then thoroughly irrigated the area with saline to look for any remaining loose fragments. We held this in place with a towel clip as we drilled a transverse hole through the ulna, perhaps 2.5 cm distal to the fracture site. We passed an 18-gauge wire through this transverse tunnel through the ulna, and then we passed two smooth Steinmann pins across the fracture site. We started the Steinmann pins from the proximal fragment and drilled across the fracture site into the distal ulnar shaft. After we had completed the second Steinmann pin across the fracture site, we passed the 18-gauge wire in a figure-of-eight fashion across the fracture site and around the Steinmann pins. We then tightened this with a Harris wire tightener. The combination of the Steinmann pins and the figure-of-eight wire seemed to secure the fracture quite nicely. There was no movement of the fracture site with placing the elbow through a range of motion. We left the Steinmann pins long until we had obtained an intraoperative x-ray confirming an acceptable alignment of the fragment. The x-rays did confirm a significant loss of the articular cartilage; however, it was elected to accept this because the fragments appeared to be relatively stable clinically.

We then bent the Steinmann pins at 90 degrees and cut them off and then taped the Steinmann pins so that they were buried into the triceps muscle. We placed the elbow through a range of motion and found that no crepitus was noted. The fracture appeared to be in good condition, and we therefore irrigated the area with saline and closed the subcutaneous tissue using 2-0 Vicryl and the skin with 3-0 nylon. A Xeroform dressing was applied, and a long-arm splint was applied with the elbow flexed about 60 degrees. He was taken from the operating room in good condition and breathing spontaneously. Tourniquet released after 43 minutes of tourniquet time, and we released this just after the x-rays. He was given IV Kefzol preoperatively and will be continued on IV Kefzol for 24 hours postoperatively as well. The final sponge and needle counts were correct.

19. OPERATIVE REPORT

PREOPERATIVE DIAGNOSIS: Left lung abscess.

POSTOPERATIVE DIAGNOSIS: Same.

PROCEDURE PERFORMED: Left upper lobectomy with decortication and drainage.

INDICATIONS: This 52-year-old female with radiographic evidence of a left upper lobe abscess was admitted the evening before surgery with tension pneumothorax treated with double-lumen intubation and a chest tube. She was subsequently dialyzed to improve hemodynamics and oxygenation and was felt to be as optimal as possible for her left thoracotomy.

FINDINGS AT SURGERY revealed a large abscess in the left upper lobe accounting for approximately 70% of the left upper lobe parenchyma. Fibrinopurulent exudate was noted on the left lower lobe and throughout the parietal pleural surfaces. This was removed piecemeal with gradual improvement in the left lower lobe pulmonary expansion.

PROCEDURE: The patient was brought to the operating room and placed in the supine position, and under general intubation with a double-lumen tube that had been placed the night before, the patient was rolled into the right lateral decubitus position with her left side up. A posterolateral thoracotomy was performed. Adhesions were taken down sharply and bluntly and with cautery. Following this, a standard artery first left upper lobectomy was carried out utilizing 0 silk and hemoclips. The left upper pulmonary vein was secured with a single application of the TA-30 vascular stapling machine. The posterior fissure was created with multiple applications of the TIA automatic stapling machine and the bronchus secured with a single application of the TA-30 bronchus stapling machine. Following this, the wound was drained with three 24-French atrium chest tubes and hemostasis obtained with spray Tisseel, Surgicel gauze. The bronchus was sealed with Bio-glue and the wound closed in layers and a sterile compression dressing applied, and the patient returned to the surgical intensive care unit after changing the double-lumen tube to a single-lumen tube. The patient received 3 units of packed cells intraoperatively to maintain hemostasis. Sponge count and needle count correct × 2.

PATHOLOGY REPORT LATER INDICATED: See Report 65.

20. OPERATIVE REPORT

Endocervical and Endometrial Biopsy

The patient is a 60-year-old married white female, whose last menstrual period was at age 55. No postmenopausal bleeding. Pap is current. Mammogram is not given.

CHIEF COMPLAINT: Metastatic clear cell carcinoma.

The patient is status post CT-guided transgluteal biopsy of a presacral mass, which returns as metastatic clear cell carcinoma. Biopsy was performed September 17, 20XX. The patient's CT of the abdomen shows the uterus to be slightly enlarged for patient's age but does not mention ascites or ovarian masses.

MEDICATIONS:

1. Citracal.
2. Lanoxin 0.25 mg.
3. Metoprolol 50 mg b.i.d.
4. Multivitamin.

5. Ocuvite.
6. Xanax.

MEDICAL PROBLEMS:

1. Chronic pelvic pain syndrome.
2. Sacroiliac lipoma.
3. Pudendal neuralgia.
4. Hiatal hernia.

FAMILY HISTORY: Negative.

REVIEW OF SYSTEMS: Positive for glasses, high blood pressure, anxiety, depression.

PROCEDURE: Endocervical and endometrial biopsy.

The patient received antibiotic prophylaxis and then the procedure was performed by visualizing the cervix. The cervix was prepped with Betadine, and cytobrush was then used to obtain cervical curetting. The endocervical os was unable to be demonstrated by the Pipelle curette or the uterine sound. The cytobrush was then used to locate the central endometrial canal, and the Pipelle curette was then used to obtain endometrial curetting. Bimanual examination shows the uterus to measure 4 to 6 weeks, anteverted, smooth, mobile. Adnexa negative. Rectal declined. BUS within normal limits.

IMPRESSION: Clear cell carcinoma of unknown origin.

PLAN: Refer the patient to the University of Minnesota for diagnostic workup and treatment. The patient and University of Minnesota will be advised of the results of the biopsies when they become available.

PATHOLOGY REPORT LATER INDICATED: See Report 54.

21. OPERATIVE REPORT

PREOPERATIVE DIAGNOSIS: Atelectasis of the right lower lobe, suspecting either a mucus plug or obstructing cancer.

POSTOPERATIVE DIAGNOSIS: Mildly inflamed airways with some thick secretions. No definite mucus plug was seen, and certainly no cancer was noted.

PROCEDURE PERFORMED: Bronchoalveolar lavage, bronchial brushings, and bronchial washings.

For a detail of drugs used and amounts of drugs used, please refer to the bronchoscopy report sheet.

The patient was in the ICU on the ventilator, intubated, and so we simply used ICU sedation. We put the bronchoscope down the endotracheal tube. We could see the trachea, which appeared okay. The carina appeared normal. In the right and left lungs, all segments were patent and entered, and in the right lower lobe and middle lower lobe, there were increased, thick, tenacious secretions. No definite mucus plug. It did take a little suctioning to dislodge all of the mucus; however, it was not as bad as I thought it would be looking at the x-ray. The area was brushed, washed, and then, to be more specific, because of evidence on chest x-ray of something going on in the periphery, a bronchoalveolar lavage of the right lower lobe is performed. The patient tolerated the procedure well. Specimens were performed. Specimens were sent for appropriate cytological, pathological, and bacteriological studies, and we hope to be able to follow up on that tomorrow.

PATHOLOGY REPORT LATER INDICATED: See Report 66.

22. OPERATIVE REPORT

PREOPERATIVE DIAGNOSIS: Chronic adenotonsillitis and chronic tonsillitis.

POSTOPERATIVE DIAGNOSIS: Chronic adenotonsillitis and chronic tonsillitis.

PROCEDURE PERFORMED: Tonsillectomy and adenoidectomy.

OPERATIVE NOTE: The patient is a 15-year-old woman who was seen in the office and diagnosed with the above condition. Decision was made in consultation with the patient to undergo the procedure.

She was admitted through the same-day department and taken to the operating room, where she was administered general anesthetic by intravenous injection. She was then intubated endotracheally. The Jennings gag was inserted into the mouth and expanded; this was secured to a Mayo stand. Two red rubber catheters were placed through the nose and brought out through the mouth; these were secured with snaps. This was done to elevate the palate. A laryngeal mirror was placed in the nasopharynx. The adenoid tissue was visualized. Using suction cautery, the adenoid tissue was removed in systemic fashion. Once this was completed, the red rubbers were released and brought out through the nose. The right tonsil was grasped with an Allis forceps and retracted medially using a harmonic scalpel, and the capsule was entered bilaterally. The tonsil was removed from its fossa in an inferior fashion, and one small area was cauterized. The left tonsil was then grasped with an Allis forceps and retracted medially. Again, the capsule was identified laterally, and the harmonic scalpel was used to remove the tonsil from its fossa in an inferior to superior fashion. Once this was completed, the bed was inspected, and two small areas were cauterized here. Three tonsillar sponges were soaked in 1% Marcaine with epinephrine; one was placed in the nasopharynx, and one in each tonsil bed. These were left in position for 5 minutes, and at the end of this interval they were removed. The beds were inspected. No further bleeding was noted. The gag was then removed from the mouth. The TMJ joint was checked. The patient was allowed to recover from a general anesthetic and taken to the post anesthesia care unit in stable condition. There were no complications during this procedure.

PATHOLOGY REPORT LATER INDICATED: Benign tonsil and adenoid tissue.

23. OPERATIVE REPORT

PREOPERATIVE DIAGNOSIS: Pleural fluid, unknown cause.

POSTOPERATIVE DIAGNOSIS: Loculated pleural effusion with removal of 40 cc of bloody pleural fluid.

PROCEDURE PERFORMED: Diagnostic thoracentesis.

On ultrasound, the areas were loculated by that method as well as by attempting to draw out fluid. I had to do four different sticks to get 40 cc of fluid and that was about the extent of each pocket. There were four different pockets I entered just in the one general area that was marked by ultrasound. This, of course, was done after marking it with ultrasound, rubbing the area with swabs to sterilize the area, and then using 20 cc of 1% lidocaine for local anesthesia. With a one-pass maneuver, we were able to get into some fluid. At first actually, we did not get any fluid. We moved over about 1 inch, and then we were able to get 10 cc of fluid before the pocket petered out. The next one we got 5 cc, and I had to go to a different pocket to get that. Then in the fourth pocket we were able to get two syringefuls with 10 cc to get at least 40 cc of fluid. As this was such a tenuous area, I did not put a chest tube in to drain it because I did not think we would get anything that would amount to anything with the small chest tube I had at my command. I think we might need thoracoscopy to break up adhesions and drain it right. Of course, the differential of bloody pleural fluid includes tuberculosis, trauma, cancer, and pulmonary embolus. A V/Q scan would probably be pointless in this particular effort. I think I would wait to see what the cultures are before I went down the pulmonary embolus tree. I will have to get ahold of Dr. Marrot about CT surgery.

PATHOLOGY REPORT LATER INDICATED: See Report 67.

24. OPERATIVE REPORT

PROCEDURE PERFORMED: Fiberoptic bronchoscopy, bronchial biopsy, bronchial washings, bronchial brushings.

PREPROCEDURE DIAGNOSIS: Abnormal chest x-ray.

POSTPROCEDURE DIAGNOSIS: Inflammation in all lobes, pneumonia. With pleural plaquing consistent with possible candidiasis.

The patient was already on a ventilator, so the bronchoscope tube was introduced through the endotracheal tube. We saw 2.5 cm above the carina of the trachea, which was red and swollen, as was the carina. The right lung—all entrances were patent, but they were all swollen and red, with increased secretions. The left lung was even more involved, with more swelling and more edema and had bloody secretions, especially at the left base. This area from the carina all the way down to the smaller airways on the left side had shown white plaquing consistent with possible candidiasis. These areas were brushed, washed, biopsied. A biopsy specimen was also sent for tissue culture, as well as two biopsy specimens sent for pathology. Sheath brushings were also performed. The patient tolerated the procedure well, was still in the ICU, monitored throughout the procedure.

25. CARDIAC CATHETERIZATION REPORT

PROCEDURES PERFORMED: Left-sided heart catheterization, selective coronary angiography, and left ventriculography.

INDICATION: Chest pain and abnormal Cardiolite stress test.

COMPLICATIONS: None.

RESULTS:

I. HEMODYNAMICS: The left ventricular pressure before the LV-gram was 117/1 with an LVEDP of 4. After the LV-gram, it was 111/4 with an LVEDP of 10. The aortic pressure on pullback was 111/17.

II. LEFT VENTRICULOGRAPHY: The left ventriculography showed that the left ventricle was of normal size. There were no significant segmental wall motion abnormalities. The overall left ventricular systolic function was normal with an ejection fraction of better than 60%.

III. SELECTIVE CORONARY ANGIOGRAPHY:

A. RIGHT CORONARY ARTERY: The right coronary artery is a medium to large size dominant artery that has about 80% to 90% proximal/mid eccentric stenosis. The rest of the artery has only mild surface irregularities. The PDA and the posterolateral branches are small in size and have only mild surface irregularities.

B. LEFT MAIN CORONARY ARTERY: The left main has mild distal narrowing.

C. LEFT CIRCUMFLEX ARTERY: The left circumflex artery was a medium size, nondominant artery. It gave rise to a very high first obtuse marginal/intermedius, which was a bifurcating medium size artery that has only mild surface irregularities. The second obtuse marginal was also a medium size artery that has about 20% to 25% proximal narrowing. After that second obtuse marginal, the circumflex artery was a small size artery that has about 20% to 30% narrowing, a small aneurysmal segment. After that, it continued as a small third obtuse marginal that has mild atherosclerotic disease.

D. LEFT ANTERIOR DESCENDING CORONARY ARTERY: The left anterior descending artery was a medium size artery that is mildly calcified. It gave rise to a very tiny first diagonal that has mild diffuse atherosclerotic disease. Right at the origin of the second diagonal, the LAD has about 30% narrowing. The rest of the artery was free of significant obstructive disease. The second diagonal was also a small caliber artery that has no significant obstructive disease.

CONCLUSION:

1. Normal overall left ventricular systolic function
2. Severe single vessel atherosclerotic heart disease

RECOMMENDATIONS: Angioplasty stent of the right coronary artery.

26. CORONARY ARTERY BYPASS SURGERY

PREOPERATIVE DIAGNOSIS: Atherosclerotic heart disease, coronary artery disease with depressed LV function.

POSTOPERATIVE DIAGNOSIS: Same.

PROCEDURE PERFORMED: Single vessel coronary artery bypass grafting, LIMA to LAD, off-pump.

ANESTHESIA: General endotracheal.

SPONGE COUNT, NEEDLE COUNT, INSTRUMENT COUNT: Correct.

ESTIMATED BLOOD LOSS: Approximately 666 cc and CellSaver given back is approximately 287 cc.

DRAINS: Four 19-French round Blake drains, one in the left chest, one in the right chest, one over the heart, and one over the pericardial wall, placed to Pleur-evac suction.

INDICATIONS: The patient is a 62-year-old man who has undergone approximately 12 heart catheterizations in the last several years. He has had recurrent in-stent stenosis of the proximal LAD lesion and also a branch of an OM with disease proximally. The patient is taken to the operating room because of recurrent angina, Class III anginal symptoms.

PROCEDURE: After informed consent was obtained, the patient was taken to the operating room. The patient was properly identified. A Swan-Ganz catheter was placed and a right arterial line was placed. A Foley catheter was inserted. The patient was prepped from his chin to both feet bilaterally. A midline sternotomy was performed. The sternum was divided with the sternal saw and the left internal mammary was harvested in a standard fashion.

Simultaneously, the right greater saphenous vein was harvested beginning in the thigh and extending down to the level of the knee. The vein was adequate for bypass grafting. It was excised. The wound was then closed in layers.

Once the LIMA was nearly completely dissected free, the patient was heparinized. The LIMA was divided distally and noted to have excellent flow. It was tied distally. LIMA bed was examined for bleeding. There appeared to be no bleeding present from the LIMA bed. Attention was then turned to the pericardium. The pericardium was opened. Pericardial stay sutures were placed. The left side of the pericardium was fashioned so that the LIMA could sit nicely to the LAD under the lung. Deep pericardial stitch was placed allowing the heart to be elevated and brought medially. A stay suture was placed around the proximal LAD and around the distal LAD. The octopus stabilizing device was used to stabilize the LAD at its mid portion. The proximal stay suture was placed down on the LAD. The LAD was opened and the LIMA had been fashioned for the anastomosis, and the LIMA to LAD anastomosis was carried out using a 7-0 Prolene in a continuous running fashion using a single knot technique. LIMA pedicle was then sutured down. There appeared to be no leak present from the LIMA anastomosis. The starfish stabilizing device was placed on the apex of the heart. The heart was elevated. The lateral wall of the heart was examined extensively for the OM branch that had some proximal disease in it. This artery was not able to be identified. The heart was covered heavily in fat, making it somewhat more difficult, but a thorough examination was carried out. At this point I actually broke scrub, went to the catheterization laboratory, re-examined the heart catheterization, and then went back to the OR again looking for that vessel. It almost could have been acting like a high diagonal vessel as it was a high OM, but again in this territory in this distribution I could not identify that vessel, so only a single vessel LIMA to LAD anastomosis was created, and the patient ended up with a single bypass. I think he should do well with just a single bypass.

The surgical sites were all examined for bleeding, and there appeared to be no bleeding present. The patient was reversed with 50 mg of Protamine and four Blake drains were placed, one in the left chest, one in the right chest, one over the heart, and one in the pericardial wall. The patient tolerated the procedure well. The preoperative and postoperative transesophageal echocardiogram looked fine. Sternal wires were placed and then the wound was closed in layers. Initial cardiac index here revealed a cardiac index of approximately 2.4 on low-dose nitro drip.

27. OPERATIVE REPORT

PREOPERATIVE DIAGNOSIS: Symptomatic right internal carotid artery stenosis.

POSTOPERATIVE DIAGNOSIS: Symptomatic right internal carotid artery stenosis.

OPERATIVE PROCEDURE:

1. Right carotid thromboendarterectomy with patch placement.
2. Intraoperative electroencephalogram monitoring.

INDICATION: This 30-year-old woman has a tight right internal carotid artery stenosis. She has had an episode of amaurosis fugax. She has some other medical problems that also complicate her overall situation, but she has a significantly tight stenosis that is symptomatic, and I would recommend an endarterectomy for this. The procedure, along with the risks, has been previously discussed with the patient. Please see the clinic notes. We will be doing this with the patient awake. We also will be doing EEG monitoring though because of the patient's overall condition, and if she does not end up needing to be intubated during the middle of the case, we will still be able to monitor her brain activity.

PROCEDURE: This was done with the patient under cervical block. Local anesthesia was also infiltrated (0.5% Marcaine with epinephrine). Dissection was carried down through a cervical oblique incision along the anterior border of the sternocleidomastoid muscle. Dissection was carried down to the carotid artery. The common carotid as well as the internal and external carotid arteries and superior thyroid arteries were all dissected free sharply and circumferentially controlled with vessel loops. The common carotid was controlled with umbilical tape and Rumel tourniquet. The patient was systemically heparinized. ACTs were obtained and followed. The ICA was occluded, then the common and then the external carotid. Arteriotomy was made. The plaque was hemorrhagic and ulcerated. It was quite friable. We were able to dissect this out with Freer elevator. This came out quite nicely. The distal endpoint feathered off nicely, but we did place one single tacking suture at the 6-o'clock position. This was 7-0 Prolene. We then used the Impra carotid patch to close the arteriotomy site. This was done with a CV-7 Gore-Tex suture in a running fashion. We heparinized, backbled, and forebled. Intermittently, we had her move her left hand during the case. After suturing the suture line, we opened up the external carotid and the common carotid. After about 10 heartbeats, we then opened up the internal carotid artery. There was bleeding from needle holes. This was controlled with FloSeal. There was good flow through all the arteries at the end of the procedure by Doppler. A 10-mm flat Jackson-Pratt drain was placed before closure of the wound. Hemostasis was present. At the end of the procedure in the admit room, she was awake and following commands and moving all of her extremities. She went to the recovery room in stable condition. I met with the patient's family postoperatively to discuss the operation.

ADDENDUM: It should be noted that this procedure was done with intraoperative EEG monitoring. No changes were noted in the EEG during the procedure. Clamp time was 40 minutes. A patch closure was used as noted. She was also reversed with 40 mg of protamine at the end of the procedure.

28. OPERATIVE REPORT

INDICATION: Prolonged fetal heart rate deceleration. *(report delivery complicated by fetal heart rate)*

PROCEDURE: Vacuum-assisted vaginal delivery. *(report delivery vacuum assisted)*

COMPLICATIONS: Shoulder dystocia, relieved with McRobert's maneuver. *(report delivery complication due to shoulder presentation)*

PREAMBLE: The patient is a 33-year-old gravida 3, para 2, 38 week, 3 days gestation, admitted from the emergency department secondary to pelvic pain *(not reported because the pain is part of delivery)*. The patient was quite uncomfortable and had artificial rupture of membranes followed by labor progression to full dilation. She then began pushing, and some prolonged fetal heart rate decelerations down to about 90 beats per minute were noted *(supports delivery complicated by fetal heart rate)*. Because of this, a decision was made to proceed with vacuum extraction *(supports delivery vacuum assisted)* to assist in expediting delivery.

PROCEDURE NOTE: Maternal bladder was emptied using straight catheter. Pelvic examination was carried out and the cervix was confirmed to be fully dilated. Fetal vertex was present at +1 station. The small kiwi cup vacuum *(supports delivery vacuum assisted)* was then applied to the fetal vertex. On the second pull, there was one pop off, but this was after good descent of the fetal head had been achieved. Baby then delivered and was a live-born male infant. There was moderate shoulder dystocia present *(supports delivery complicated by shoulder presentation)* and this was relieved with McRobert's maneuver. The baby was handed off to the NICU team and is currently in the NICU for further observation. Apgar's *(a newborn maturity scoring method)* are not available at this time. Cord blood gas is also pending. After an episiotomy, a second-degree perineal tear still occurred during delivery. This was repaired using 3-0 chromic in usual manner. The patient tolerated this procedure well. Estimated blood loss during delivery was 200 cc.

29. OPERATIVE REPORT

PREOPERATIVE DIAGNOSES:

1. Intrauterine pregnancy, 39 weeks.
2. Multiparity.
3. Desires permanent sterilization.
4. History of previous cesarean section × 2.

POSTOPERATIVE DIAGNOSES:

1. Intrauterine pregnancy, 39 weeks.
2. Multiparity.
3. Desires permanent sterilization.
4. History of previous cesarean section × 2.

PROCEDURE: Repeat low transverse cervical segment cesarean section with postpartum tubal ligation.

ANESTHESIA: Spinal.

ESTIMATED BLOOD LOSS: 800 cc

URINE OUTPUT: 40 cc

FLUIDS: 3000 cc

COMPLICATIONS: None.

FINDINGS: Viable male infant *(report the outcome of delivery)* weighing 6 pounds 10 ounces with Apgar's of 9 at 1 minute and 10 at 5 minutes.

PROCEDURE: The patient was prepped and draped in a supine position with left lateral displacement of the uterine fundus. Under spinal anesthesia and Foley catheter indwelling, a transverse incision was made in the lower abdomen using the old scar. The fascia was divided laterally. Rectus muscles were divided in the midline. The peritoneum was entered in a sharp manner. The incision was extended vertically. The bladder flap was created using sharp and blunt dissection and reflected inferiorly. The uterus was entered in a sharp manner in the lower uterine segment, and the incision was extended laterally with blunt traction. The head was delivered, the infant was delivered, and the infant was bulb suctioned while the cord was being doubly clamped and divided. The infant was given to the intensive care nursery staff in good condition. The placenta was manually expressed. Uterus was delivered through the abdominal cavity and placed on a wet lap sponge. A dry lap sponge was used to ensure that the remaining products of conception were removed. The cervical os was ensured patent with a ring forceps. The uterus incision was closed with 0 Vicryl in an interlocking suture in two layers with second layer imbricating the first. Figure-of-eight sutures were also placed as required for hemostasis. Operative site was inspected, irrigated, and hemostatic. The bladder flap was reapproximated using 2-0 Vicryl in a continuous suture in the midline. The left tube was identified in its entirety, including the fimbriated end and was grasped at its midportion and elevated. The mesosalpinx was transected using the Bovie. Approximately 3 cm of tube was isolated and excised. The proximal end of the distal portion and the distal end of the proximal portion were ligated with 0 chromic suture. The right tube was identified and ligated in the same fashion. Operative site was inspected and was hemostatic. Uterus was placed back in the midabdominal cavity. Pelvic gutters were irrigated. The anterior peritoneum was reapproximated with 2-0 Vicryl continuous suture. The incision was irrigated. Subcutaneous drain was placed, and the skin was closed with 2-0 silk. Sponges and needles were accounted for at the completion of the procedure. The patient left the operating room in apparent good condition after tolerating the procedure well. The Foley catheter was patent and draining a small amount of clear urine at the completion of the procedure.

30. OPERATIVE REPORT

PREOPERATIVE DIAGNOSIS: Complicated pregnancy with prior cesarean sections.

POSTOPERATIVE DIAGNOSIS: Complicated pregnancy with prior cesarean sections. *(Z code for history of obstetrical disorder affecting management of current pregnancy)*

PROCEDURE PERFORMED: Amniocentesis for fetal lung maturity.

INDICATIONS: The patient is at 38½-weeks' gestation and has had three prior C-sections and hospitalizations for recurrent episodes of pyelonephritis. *(Z code for personal history a specified urinary system disorder)* We desired to check fetal maturity so we could expedite delivery if possible.

PROCEDURE: The patient was scanned with ultrasound, and few pockets of amniotic fluid were noted; therefore we elected to do a suprapubic tap. The abdomen was prepped and draped. Dr. Marco elevated the breech of the infant up out of the pelvis, and we scanned suprapubically and found a nice pocket of amniotic fluid. A single tap was done and 10 cc of clear yellow fluid obtained. This fluid was checked for pH and was deeply blue on Nitrazine, indicating it to be most likely amniotic fluid, not urine. She tolerated this well.

Cytology report later indicated slightly decreased fetal lung maturity based on levels of phosphatidylglycerol, with recommendation to re-evaluate in 10 days. *(abnormal amnion, affecting fetus)*

31. OPERATIVE REPORT

Colonoscopy and Polypectomy

PREOPERATIVE DIAGNOSIS: Hematochezia.

POSTOPERATIVE DIAGNOSIS: Two small polyps in the cecum ascending colon, hot biopsied off. A small rectal polyp, hot biopsied off.

INDICATION: This is a 46-year-old white male with Tourette's and some MR who has had some hematochezia. There are no risk factors with no other symptoms.

PREOPERATIVE MEDICATIONS: Fentanyl 100 mcg IV; Versed 4 mg IV.

FINDINGS: The Pentax video colonoscope was inserted without difficulty to the cecum. The ileocecal valve was identified. The appendiceal orifice was seen. I could not enter the cecum. Just above the valve, there was a small 2- to 3-cm polyp. This was hot biopsied off. There was a sessile 3-mm polyp in the proximal ascending colon, hot biopsied off. Inspection of the remainder of the ascending colon, hepatic flexure, transverse colon, splenic flexure, descending colon, and sigmoid colon, revealed no erythema, ulceration, exudate, friability, or other mucosal abnormalities. The rectum showed a small 2-mm polyp that was hot biopsied off. The patient tolerated the procedure well.

IMPRESSION: Three small polyps, two in the cecum ascending colon area and one on the rectum, hot biopsied off.

PLAN: If these polyps are adenomatous, the patient should return again in 5 years for surveillance.

PATHOLOGY REPORT LATER INDICATED: See Report 56.

32. OPERATIVE REPORT

PREOPERATIVE DIAGNOSIS: Nonhealing duodenal ulcer.

POSTOPERATIVE DIAGNOSIS: Nonhealing duodenal ulcer.

PROCEDURES PERFORMED:

1. Exploratory laparotomy.
2. Partial gastrectomy (antrectomy).
3. Truncal vagotomy.
4. Gastrojejunostomy.
5. Cholecystectomy with intraoperative cholangiogram.

INDICATION: The patient is a 60-year-old female who presented with a nonhealing gastric ulcer. She has had symptoms for about a year. She complains of epigastric pain. Medical therapy with Prilosec failed, as did therapy for *H. pylori*. Biopsy of the ulcer has been done, and it was benign. The patient had a negative workup for gastrinoma. Calcium level was also normal. The patient now presents for exploratory laparotomy and partial gastrectomy. The risks and benefits were discussed with the patient in detail. She understood and agreed to proceed.

PROCEDURE: The patient was brought to the operating room. Her abdomen was prepped and draped in a sterile fashion. A midline umbilical incision was made. The peritoneal cavity was entered. Initial inspection of the peritoneal cavity showed normal liver, spleen, colon, and small bowel. There was an ulcer along the first portion of the duodenum just beyond the pylorus with some scarring. There was also an ulcer in the posterior part of the duodenal bulb, which was penetrating to the pancreas. We started dissection along the greater curvature of the stomach. Vessels were ligated with 2-0 silk ties. There was an enlarged lymph node along the greater curvature of the stomach, which was sent for frozen section. It proved to be a benign lymph node. This was the only enlarged node found during dissection. We then proceeded with truncal vagotomy. The anterior vagus and posterior vagus were identified. They were clipped proximally and distally, and a segment of each nerve was excised and sent for frozen section, and a segment of both vagus nerves was excised and confirmed by frozen section. An incision was made around the gastrohepatic ligament. The mesentery along the lesser curvature of the stomach was dissected. The vessels were ligated with 2-0 silk ties along the lesser curvature of the stomach. A Kocher maneuver was performed to aid mobilization. The pancreas was completely normal. No masses were found in the pancreas. There was penetration of the ulcer in the superior part of the head of the pancreas. Dissection was continued posterior to the stomach. The adhesions posterior to the stomach were taken down. The ulcer was in the posterior segment of the duodenal bulb just beyond the pylorus and it had penetrated the pancreas. All the posterior layer of the ulcer that was left adherent to the pancreas was shaved off. The stomach was divided with the GIA stapler so that the complete antrum would be in the specimen. The duodenum was divided between clamps. The stomach pylorus and first part of the duodenum were sent to pathology for examination. Then the duodenal stump was closed with running suture. Using 3-0 Lembert sutures, the posterior wall of the ulcer was incorporated for duodenal closure. The base of the duodenum was rolled over the ulcer, and it was all-incorporating to the duodenal closure. Our next step was to proceed with cholecystectomy. The gallbladder was separated from the liver, reflected, and taken down, and the gallbladder was divided from the liver with blunt dissection and cautery. The cystic artery was doubly ligated with silk. The cystic duct was identified. The cystic duct and gallbladder junction and gallbladder ducts were identified. Intraoperative cholangiogram was performed showing free flow of bile into the intrahepatic duct and into the duodenum. No leaks were seen. The cystic duct was doubly ligated, and the gallbladder was sent to pathology. The staple line in the proximal stomach was oversewn with 3-0 silk Lembert sutures. A retrocolic isoperistaltic Hofmeister-type gastrojejunostomy was performed on the remaining stomach and loop of jejunum. This was an isoperistaltic end-to-side two-layer anastomosis with 3-0 chromic and 3-0 silk. The stomach was secured to the transverse mesocolon with several interrupted silk sutures to prevent any herniation along the retrocolic space.

The anastomosis had a good lumen and good blood supply. There was no twist along the anastomosis. Before the anastomosis was finished, a nasogastric tube was placed along the afferent limb of the jejunum to decompress the duodenum and prevent blow out of the duodenal stump. Extra holes were made in the NG tube to provide adequate drainage. The anastomosis was marked with two clips on each side, and a Jackson-Pratt drain was placed over the duodenal stump. The peritoneal cavity was irrigated until clear. Hemostasis was adequate. The fascia was then closed with interrupted 0 Ethibond sutures. Skin edges were approximated with staples. Subcutaneous tissues were irrigated before closure. Estimated blood loss throughout the procedure was 200 ml. IV fluids: 3400 ml. Urine output: 840 ml.

FINDINGS:

1. Nonhealing benign ulcer in the posterior duodenal bulb penetrating into the head of the pancreas.
2. Partial gastrectomy *(antrectomy performed)* and excision of the pylorus, first portion of the duodenum along with ulcer.
3. Hofmeister-type retrocolic isoperistaltic gastrojejunostomy.
4. Posterior wall of the ulcer that was penetrating into the pancreas incorporated into closure of the duodenal stump.
5. Truncal vagotomy performed with intraoperative frozen section confirming both vagus nerves.
6. Cholecystectomy performed due to chronic cholecystitis with normal intraoperative cholangiogram.
7. Jackson-Pratt drain placed over the duodenal stump.

The items that are to be coded are listed below:

Partial gastrectomy *(antrectomy)* with gastrojejunostomy
Truncal vagotomy
Cholecystectomy with intraoperative cholangiogram

PATHOLOGY REPORT LATER INDICATED: Tissue showed no evidence of carcinoma. The radiologist reported the x-ray with 74300.

33. OPERATIVE REPORT

PREOPERATIVE DIAGNOSIS: Fournier's gangrene.

POSTOPERATIVE DIAGNOSIS: Fournier's gangrene, gastric foreign bodies.

PROCEDURES PERFORMED:

1. Exploratory laparotomy with gastrotomy and removal of gastric foreign body.
2. Placement of 18-French Moss gastrojejunostomy feeding tube.
3. Diverting end-sigmoid colostomy *(Hartmann's procedure)*.

ANESTHESIA: General.

INDICATIONS: This is a 33-year-old patient with Fournier's gangrene who presents today for a diverting colostomy due to wound care and placement of a gastrostomy tube for help with further follow-up feeding. He presents today for exploration. The family understands the risks of bleeding, infection, and postoperative fluid collections and wishes to proceed.

PROCEDURE: The patient was brought to the operating room, placed under general anesthesia, and prepped and draped with Betadine solution. A midline incision was made with a #10 blade and dissection was carried down through subcutaneous tissues using electrocautery. The midline fascia was identified and divided. The posterior sheath and peritoneum were sharply incised, thus allowing entry into the peritoneal cavity. There was some free fluid within the peritoneal cavity but no evidence of any abnormalities. We first identified the stomach and could feel what we felt were some polyps in the stomach. We first placed concentric purse-string sutures along the greater curvature of the stomach, opened up the stomach, and then passed an 18-French Moss gastrojejunostomy tube but were unable to get it down through the pylorus. We could feel these multiple masses in the stomach. We tied the purse-string sutures and inflated the balloon. We then made a small opening in the stomach with electrocautery and retrieved about 20 large what appeared to be vegetable matter and partially digested peppers and pickles. We irrigated with saline and then were able to pass the Moss gastrojejunostomy tube, the distal end, down through the pylorus. We closed the gastrotomy with a running 3-0 Vicryl and an outer layer of 3-0 silk Lembert sutures. We irrigated this area well. We then identified the sigmoid colon, fired a TLC-75 stapler across the sigmoid/descending colon, and then placed a 3-0 Prolene on the rectal stump. We divided the mesentery between right angle clamps and tied the pedicles with 3-0 silk ties. We had a previously marked stomal opening in the left lower quadrant. We grasped this with a Kocher clamp, made an elliptical incision around this, and then divided the anterior sheath of the rectus in cruciate fashion, divided through the rectus muscles, and then opened the posterior sheath and peritoneum. We brought the colon then through this area. There was good mobility of the colon, and the colon was viable. We then irrigated the abdomen with saline, and, once all sponge and needle counts were correct, we closed the midline fascia with a combination of interrupted 0 Vicryl and running 0 PDS. The skin was closed with skin clips. The staple line was then removed from the colon and the colostomy was matured with 3-0 Vicryl sutures. An appliance was placed. All sponge and needle counts were correct. He tolerated this well.

Prior to leaving the operating room, we took down the dressings of his right leg. There was good granulation tissue, which was pink and viable, and we then re-dressed the wound and sent him back to the surgical critical care unit in critical but stable condition.

PATHOLOGY REPORT LATER INDICATED: Idiopathic gangrene. Numerous undigested vegetable matter.

34. OPERATIVE REPORT

PREOPERATIVE DIAGNOSIS: Severe internal and external hemorrhoids.

POSTOPERATIVE DIAGNOSIS: Same.

PROCEDURE PERFORMED: Three quadrant hemorrhoidectomy.

ANESTHESIA: Spinal.

INDICATION: This is a very pleasant female who presents today with severe internal and external hemorrhoids for elective excision. She understands the risks of bleeding, infection, and postoperative fluid collection. She wishes to proceed.

PROCEDURE: The patient was brought to the operating room and placed under spinal anesthesia, prepped, and draped sterilely with Betadine solution. Digital rectal examination was first performed. There were severe external hemorrhoids. Pratt anoscope was inserted. The severest of the hemorrhoids were at the 6-o'clock, 9-o'clock, and 3-o'clock positions. These were each grasped with an Allis clamp, excised in diamond shape fashion. The mucosal defects were closed with running locked 3-0 Vicryl with the suture lines imbricated with 3-0 chromic sutures. This gave us a good closure that was hemostatic. We anesthetized the area with 30 cc of 0.5% Sensorcaine with epinephrine solution and then placed four gauze in the rectal canal. She tolerated this well and was taken to recovery in stable condition.

PATHOLOGY REPORT LATER INDICATED: Benign tissue.

35. OPERATIVE REPORT

PROCEDURE: Placement of CORFLO, feeding tube.

INDICATION: Feeding, patient with gastroparesis.

PROCEDURE: The patient was placed in the sitting position and then tilted to the right with a wedge. CORFLO was placed at the level of 19 cm without any complications. KUB was then done demonstrating the tip of the CORFLO in the third portion of the duodenum. After confirmation of postpyloric position of the CORFLO, the patient was started on Ultracal at 10 cc/hr.

36. OPERATIVE REPORT

PREOPERATIVE DIAGNOSES:

1. Expressed desire of the operating gynecologist to insert indwelling ureteral stents for ease of dissection of the anticipated enlarged adherent uterus.
2. Gynecologic diagnosis of pelvic endometriosis.

POSTOPERATIVE DIAGNOSES: Same.

PROCEDURE PERFORMED: Cystourethroscopy, insertion of bilateral ureteral catheters.

PROCEDURE: After general anesthesia and after the abdomen and genitalia had been prepped and draped in the usual fashion, the patient was placed in the dorsolithotomy position. The genitalia were examined and proved to be essentially unremarkable. The urethra was instrumented with a 24-French panendoscope sheath, and, using the foroblique and right-angle lenses, inspection of the entire vesical cavity showed no indication of any pathologic lesion. There is slight indention and some of the bladder incident to the uterine impression. The two ureteral orifices appear to be essentially unremarkable. The left ureteral orifice was catheterized with a 6-French Whistle Tip catheter with ease. The catheter was advanced to approximately 25 cm on the left side. Attention was then directed to the right side, and the right ureteral orifice was catheterized with a 6-French Whistle Tip catheter. The catheter was placed at approximately 24 cm. The bladder was then entered, Panendoscope sheath was withdrawn. An 18-French 5-ml balloon Foley catheter was then inserted into the bladder and left indwelling to the Foley catheter. The two ureteral catheters were anchored with no. 1 black silk. The two ureteral catheters and the Foley catheters were then connected to straight drainage and the patient was removed from the dorsolithotomy position. Dr. Weasly, the patient's gynecologist, then proceeded with a total abdominal hysterectomy and bilateral salpingo-oophorectomy.

37. OPERATIVE REPORT

PREOPERATIVE DIAGNOSIS: Recurrent transitional cell carcinoma of the bladder.

POSTOPERATIVE DIAGNOSIS: Same.

PROCEDURE PERFORMED: Cystoscopy; multiple random bladder biopsies.

CLINICAL NOTE: This patient has recurrent transitional cell carcinoma of the bladder. He has had BCG bladder instillation to help prevent recurrence. His last instillation was 6 weeks ago. The patient is doing well. He denied any complaints.

PROCEDURE: The patient was given a general endotracheal anesthetic and prepped and draped in lithotomy position. A 24-French resectoscope was passed into the bladder under direct vision. The urethra was normal. Prostate was nonobstructed. Inspection of the bladder demonstrated areas of hyperemia that would be most consistent with BCG changes but might also represent recurrent TCC. These areas were biopsied using a cold-cup biopsy. A 24-French resectoscope loupe was then used to cauterize these areas. Ureteric orifices were identified. Clear urine could be seen effluxing bilaterally.

The patient tolerated the procedure well. A B&O suppository was placed rectally after the end of the procedure. An 18-French Foley catheter was placed to straight drainage. Bimanual examination showed no significant abnormality and the prostate felt normal.

The patient will be scheduled for recheck cystoscopy in 3 months' time providing pathology shows no evidence of recurrent tumor.

ADDENDUM: Total resected and fulgurated area of the bladder was 7 square centimeters.

PATHOLOGY REPORT LATER INDICATED: See Report 55.

38. OPERATIVE REPORT

PREOPERATIVE DIAGNOSIS: Urinary incontinence.

POSTOPERATIVE DIAGNOSIS: Same.

PROCEDURE PERFORMED: Insertion of double cuff artificial urinary sphincter with 25 cc reservoir (multicomponent).

CLINICAL NOTE: This patient has had radiation for prostate cancer. This recurred. He then had cryotherapy. His PSA is undetectable but he has significant urinary incontinence unresponsive to pharmacotherapy. External clamp devices have been unsatisfactory.

PROCEDURE NOTE: The patient was given a spinal anesthetic, prepped and draped in a supine position. A penoscrotal incision was made. A 16-French Foley was placed in the bladder to straight drainage. The urethra was dissected to the level of the bulb. The bulbocavernosus muscle was very atrophic and was not dissected off the urethra. A double cuff placement was selected. The urethra was mobilized in two places with a small bridge of tissue between them. These cuffs were incised. Both were incised at 4.5 cm. A reservoir space was created by manual dissection in the left inguinal canal into the retropubic space. The reservoir was placed, cycled, and filled with 25 cc of sterile saline. Both cuffs were placed in the usual fashion. The pump was then placed in the mid-scrotal pouch. Connections were made using a Y connector and straight connectors in the usual fashion. The system was cycled; it worked well. Foley catheter was withdrawn to insure cycling appropriately. Subcutaneous tissues were closed with 3-0 chromic and skin with a 4-0 subcuticular Vicryl stitch. The pump was cycled again and then deactivated; the Foley catheter replaced. The patient tolerated the procedure well and was transferred to the recovery room in good condition. The wounds were thoroughly irrigated with Bacitracin solution.

39. OPERATIVE REPORT

PREOPERATIVE DIAGNOSIS: Morbid obesity.

POSTOPERATIVE DIAGNOSIS: Same.

PROCEDURES:

1. Laparoscopic Roux-en-Y gastrointestinal bypass.
2. Liver biopsy.

ANESTHESIA: General.

INDICATION: The patient is a 36-year-old female who presents with morbid obesity, with a current BMI of 46.0. She has gone to the seminars, and we have discussed laparoscopic Roux-en-Y gastrointestinal bypass along with the risk of surgery including bleeding, infection, leakage from the anastomoses, conversion to open procedure, postoperative stenoses of the anastomoses, or bowel obstruction. She understands and wishes to proceed.

PROCEDURE: The patient was brought to the operating room and placed under general anesthesia. A Foley catheter and orogastric tubes were inserted. She was prepped and draped sterilely with Betadine solution. A supraumbilical incision was made with a #15 blade, and dissection was carried down through the subcutaneous tissues bluntly. The patient had an incisional hernia from an old trocar port site. We placed our operative trocar into the abdomen, insufflated the abdomen. There was no damage to the underlying viscera. Under direct vision, we then placed two, midclavicular line, 12-millimeter ports that were just lateral and above the umbilical port. There was a right upper quadrant 12-millimeter port in the anterior axillary line and a left upper quadrant 5-millimeter port in the anterior axillary line. These were all placed under direct vision with no damage to the bowel. The patient had some adhesions of her gastrohepatic ligament to the liver. We took these down using the harmonic scalpel. Before continuing, a needle specimen was obtained from the liver, appropriately marked for pathologic evaluation. We then entered the retrogastric space and placed our taut catheter behind the stomach. We then flipped the omentum up over the top of itself. We elevated the transverse colon and opened the transverse colon where we could see the drain. We identified the ligament of Treitz and fired an Endo-GIA stapler across the bowel, down from the ligament of Treitz. We fired an additional load across the mesentery. We then counted out 100 centimeters of bowel and then performed a stapled side-to-side functional end-to-end anastomosis by opening the bowel on the proximal and distal sides with the harmonic scalpel, firing two loads of the Endo-GIA stapler and closing the anastomosis with an Endo-GIA fired staple line. This gave us a nice anastomosis. We closed the mesenteric defect here with an Ethibond suture and fixed with Laparoties. We then sutured the proximal end to the catheter and flipped the mesentery back down. We then brought the bowel and the catheter up in retrogastric fashion. Next, we identified the angle of His. We opened the angle of His, and we fired five loads of the Endo-GIA stapler across the stomach. We had blown up the 20-cc balloon and had about a 20-cc pouch. Once we had completely transected the stomach, we went above and placed the Bioenteric catheter within the gastric pouch. We passed the snare through it. We made a separate stab incision in the upper abdomen and passed the wire through. We then fed the anvil end of the CEA-21 stapler down through the back of the pharynx down through the esophagus and brought out through our gastric pouch. We then enlarged the left midclavicular line, abdominal port, and placed the CEA-25 stapler through here. We opened the staple line on the bowel that we had brought up after we had removed the taut catheter and placed the CEA stapler into the bowel, brought the spike through, connected the two ends of the CEA, closed it, and fired it. This gave us a nice 21-millimeter circular anastomosis. We completed the anastomosis with the Endo-GIA stapler. We imbricated the staple line with two Ethibond sutures, placed a wad of fat over the last to adhere the fat near our staple line. We tested the anastomosis with air with the bowel clamped, and there was no evidence of a leak. We then placed Hemaseel over this anastomosis, and then once again mobilized the mesentery. We then closed the mesenteric defect where the small bowel had gone in retrogastric fashion with the Ethicon Endo-suture. We once again placed Hemaseel on our small anastomosis. We placed 10 flat Jackson-Pratt drains near our GJ anastomosis, which came on out the left side. We removed the trocar ports under direct vision. We then extended our umbilical incision and reduced the umbilical hernia. We closed the fascial defect with interrupted 0 Prolene sutures. We anesthetized the wounds at all areas with a total of 60 cc of 0.50% Sensorcaine with epinephrine solution. We secured the drains in place with 0 silk sutures and then closed the skin with 3-0 Prolene sutures. Steri-Strips and sterile Band-Aids were applied. All sponge and needle counts were correct. We left the taut catheter and a Penrose drain in the left midclavicular line incision.

All sponge and needle counts were correct. She tolerated this well and was taken to recovery in stable condition.

PATHOLOGY REPORT LATER INDICATED: See Report 63.

40. OPERATIVE REPORT

HISTORY: This patient, who is unknown to me, reports working in the shop at his home grinding metal approximately 5 hours ago. He was wearing safety glasses, but he has noticed a foreign body in his right eye. He reports slight irritation to the eye. Denies blurred vision.

PHYSICAL EXAMINATION: PERLA, fundi without edema. There was no foreign body on lid eversion. Slit lamp shows a foreign body approximately 2 to 3 o'clock on the edge of the cornea. This foreign body appears metallic. There is very small area of rust around the site. Iris is intact. There are no cells in the anterior chamber. Fluorescein dye reveals uptake only over foreign body.

PROCEDURE: Two drops of Alcaine were used in the right eye. Foreign body was removed with an eye spud without difficulty. Slight orange discoloration at the base of cornea, but no definite rust ring visible.

IMPRESSION: Residual corneal abrasion.

DISPOSITION: Foreign body removed from right eye.

41. OPERATIVE REPORT

PREOPERATIVE DIAGNOSIS: Left cervical spondylosis, C5–6, C6–7, with cervical discs.

POSTOPERATIVE DIAGNOSIS: Same.

PROCEDURE PERFORMED: Anterior discectomy and osteophytectomy for decompression at C5–6 and C6–7, with allograft fusion and Zephyr plating.

This case was monitored with sensory evoked potentials throughout the case. There were no changes.

PROCEDURE: Under general anesthesia, the patient was placed in the cervical outrigger. The neck was prepped and draped in the usual manner. An incision was made parallel to the sternocleidomastoid, and then we got onto the omohyoid and incised this. Then with sharp dissection we got onto the prevertebral fascia, put the Farley-Thompson retractor in, and then I was able to localize the C5–6 and C6–7 interspaces. The plan here was to decompress the nerve roots and get rid of the ridges, the disc, and to fuse and plate. The discectomies were done at C5–6 and C6–7. The ridges were removed, the discs were removed, and then the cartilaginous surfaces were prepared for reception of the bony fusion. At C6–7, a #8 trial was utilized and at C5–6 a #7 trial was utilized with bone. I took off the ridges, I took off the osteophytes, I removed the discs. I got down to the dura on both sides and was satisfied now that the nerve roots were decompressed and I could put the trial in and place the structural bone graft in. This was done at both levels. This having been done, they were countersunk and I then utilized a Zephyr plate from C5 down to C7 and put a screw into C6 as well. This done, a Hemovac drain was placed into the wound. Of course, the plate was locked, and we then closed the wound in layers utilizing 2-0 chromic on the platysma with 2-0 plain in the subcutaneous tissue and 3-0 nylon interrupted mattress sutures on the skin. A dressing was applied. The patient was to wear a collar in the postop period.

PATHOLOGY REPORT LATER INDICATED: Benign bone and tissue.

42. OPERATIVE REPORT

PREOPERATIVE DIAGNOSES:

1. Ptosis, mechanical, right upper lid.
2. Loss of superior visual field secondary to #1.
3. Superior hemianopia secondary to #l, right eye.

POSTOPERATIVE DIAGNOSES: Same.

PROCEDURE PERFORMED: Fasanella-Servat procedure, right upper lid.

ANESTHESIA: General endotracheal.

INDICATIONS: This 57-year-old white female has had progressively drooping lid on her right for many years from the weight of excess skin which has now reduced her superior visual field in the right eye and has actually limited her vision. After the prior approval and the photos and documentation were obtained, it was noted that the patient did have a 3- to 4-mm ptosis of the right upper lid and we would approach this with a Fasanella-Servat procedure. The risk of infection, hemorrhage, and reoperations were discussed.

PROCEDURE: After the patient was placed under suitable general endotracheal anesthesia, the superior tarsal border was then marked with a marking pen and a 15 Bard-Parker blade cut down through skin to the muscle area. The lid was then everted on a Desmarres retractor and two curved mosquitos were then placed with the point central and pointing superiorly when the lid was everted. A 6-0 gut rapid absorbing suture was then started through the skin incision at the superior tarsal border and then a purse string was then woven along the curve tips and then the 3 to 4 mm resection was then obtained and then the serpentine 6-0 gut suture was then approximated without cutting it and brought out through the skin and tied. It was allowed to retract into the knot. There was no bleeding and there was no cut suture. Maxitrol ointment, a Telfa pad, and patch was applied and the patient was sent to the recovery room. There were no complications.

43. OPERATIVE REPORT

PREOPERATIVE DIAGNOSIS: Lumbar radiculopathy secondary to herniated L5-S1 disc.

POSTOPERATIVE DIAGNOSIS: Same.

PROCEDURE PERFORMED: Right L5-S1 hemilaminectomy with excision of herniated L5-S1 disc.

PROCEDURE: The patient was taken to the operating room and placed under general endotracheal anesthesia. He was rotated into the prone position on chest rolls with arms extended over the head. The lumbar region was shaved, prepped, and draped in the usual sterile manner. The proposed vertical midline incision was infiltrated with lidocaine, with epinephrine. The skin was incised and sharp dissection carried through the subcutaneous tissues. The fascia was incised and subperiosteal dissection undertaken at L5-S1. The hemilamina of L5 was then removed in piecemeal fashion. This allowed evaluation of both the L4-5 disc as well as the L5-S1 disc. At L5-S1, moderate-sized disc herniation was immediately evident. The surrounding capsule was incised, and a large fragment of ligamentous degenerative disc was removed. The interspace was then probed, and all degenerative disc material was removed. On completion, the thecal sac and nerve root were noted to be well decompressed at L4-5. The L4-5 level appeared normal. Epidural space was lined with Surgicel and fat graft, and the wound closed in interrupted layers, with 4-0 Vicryl subcuticular stitch for skin. Steri-Strips and sterile dressing were applied to the wound. The patient tolerated the procedure well and was transferred to the recovery room in good condition.

PATHOLOGY REPORT LATER INDICATED: See Report 57.

44. OPERATIVE REPORT

PREOPERATIVE DIAGNOSES:

1. Left orbitonasal mass.
2. Dry eye syndrome.
3. Pseudophakia, both eyes.
4. Computerized tomography confirmed tumor left orbital, left nasal side.

POSTOPERATIVE DIAGNOSES: Same with the addition of low-grade lymphoma, left orbit.

PROCEDURE: Anterior orbitotomy, debulking and biopsy.

ANESTHESIA: General endotracheal anesthesia.

INDICATION: This 81-year-old white woman has had a progressively enlarging mass of the left superior nasal orbit, which had become quite hard and is attached to the bone. CT shows there has been no bony invasion, and the brain has not been invaded. More than likely, this is a lymphoma, but we want to take the patient for an anterior orbitotomy for debulking and biopsy.

DESCRIPTION OF PROCEDURE: After the patient was prepped and draped in the usual sterile fashion for ophthalmic surgery, the superior sulcus fold was marked out on her medial left upper lid. This was then cut through skin and muscle with the 25 Bard-Parker blade down through the orbital fat pad. It was noted there was some saponified fat and a hard mass that was kind of an orangish-red color and was attached to this. Two specimens were removed and tagged and sent for frozen section, and into the cryo unit with liquid nitrogen down to –80 degrees and was then brought in to remove the rest of the mass. There were some fragments of mass still attached to the nasal wall of the orbit. The frozen section revealed lymphoma, low grade, probably stage I, and since this is radiosensitive and that all of the tumor could not be removed without exenterating the orbit, it was elected to close at this point and treat the rest conservatively. The wound was closed after the remaining tumor was infiltrated with Solu-Medrol 125 mg per ml for a total of 2 ml, after which the wound was closed with interrupted 6-0 black nylon suture and Maxitrol ointment. Telfa pad, patch and shield were applied. The patient was sent to the recovery room. There were no complications.

PATHOLOGY REPORT LATER INDICATED: Lymphoma.

45. RADIOLOGY REPORT

EXAMINATION OF: Chest.

CLINICAL SYMPTOMS: Chest pain.

PORTABLE CHEST, AP SITTING (ONE VIEW), 4:45 PM: Comparisons are made with the previous study of 08/23/XX. The cardiac silhouette is not grossly enlarged for this projection. The mediastinum is not widened. Lung fields are generally clear and expanded to the periphery. Cardiac monitors do superimpose the chest.

CONCLUSION: Generally stable appearance of the chest, unchanged compared with the previous study.

46. RADIOLOGY REPORT

EXAMINATION OF: Biophysical profile.

CLINICAL SYMPTOMS: High blood pressure, estimated gestational age 28 weeks 5 days.

BIOPHYSICAL PROFILE: The placenta is located along the anterior wall. It is heterogeneous in echotexture, grade II. The AFI is 5.4 cm, which is low. Fetal motion noted by the technologist. Heart rate 147 beats per minute. Intrauterine hypoechoic area seen anteriorly within the uterus measures about 2 cm in size and a second similar-sized hypoechoic area is located within the uterus. Both findings are presumed fibroids.

They are nonspecific findings, however. Biophysical profile was scored a perfect 8 out of 8.

47. CT SCAN

EXAMINATION OF: CT of orbits.

CLINICAL SYMPTOMS: Left eye pain.

CT OF ORBITS: CT of orbits in axial and coronal planes without contrast. Patient was vomiting, therefore contrast was not given.

1. Complete opacification of right aspect of sphenoid sinus.
2. Near complete opacification of right maxillary antrum.
3. Polypoid membrane thickening left maxillary antrum.
4. Scattered membrane thickening throughout a few ethmoidal air cells.
5. Remainder negative.

48. MRA REPORT

EXAMINATION OF: MRA brain.

CLINICAL SYMPTOMS: Third nerve palsy, complete.

MAGNETIC RESONANCE EXAMINATION OF THE ARTERIAL VASCULATURE OF THE POSTERIOR FOSSA AND CIRCLE OF WILLIS REGION was performed utilizing three-dimensional time-of-flight multislab technique. Raw data and selected maximum-intensity projection images were photographed. Additionally, I have personally manipulated the maximum-intensity projections on a computer console in order to view the vasculature from various angulations.

I don't appreciate evidence of aneurysm. In particular, I don't appreciate evidence of aneurysm in the region of the posterior communicating arteries. I have personally reviewed the raw data images.

Bilaterally, there is some signal loss at the origin of the A1 segment of each anterior cerebral artery. This gives the appearance of stenosis. Most probably, this is technical, rather than due to true stenosis, but stenosis is not ruled out.

Internal carotid arteries appear unremarkable. Vertebral arteries are unremarkable. The basilar artery is unremarkable.

Proximal segments of the middle and posterior cerebral arteries appear unremarkable. Posterior communicating arteries are not visualized and are most probably very small.

49. RADIOLOGY REPORT

EXAMINATION OF: X-Ray abdomen; single view.

CLINICAL SYMPTOMS: Malnutrition.

FINDINGS: A single supine view of the abdomen is submitted for interpretation. The majority of the pelvis and a portion of the left side of the abdomen are excluded from this examination. Feeding tube is identified. The tip overlies the left upper quadrant. Air is present within both small and large bowel, which does not appear distended as visualized on this examination. There is degenerative change and dextroscoliosis of the lumbar spine. Surgical clips overlie the right upper quadrant. Opacity is noted in the left lung base, which may relate to atelectasis or infiltrate. Follow-up is suggested.

50. RADIOLOGY REPORT

EXAMINATION OF: Left foot.

CLINICAL SYMPTOMS: Severe foot pain.

TWO VIEWS, LEFT FOOT: Comparison is made with the most recent films available 10/15/XX. There is diffuse demineralization of the osseous structures of the foot. Soft-tissue swelling is seen. Erosive changes have been previously described involving multiple metatarsophalangeal joints, and these are identified once again today. The differential is not significantly changed compared with the previous examination.

IMPRESSION:

1. Overall there is no significant interval change compared with 10/15/XX. There are extensive demineralization and extensive erosive changes involving the metatarsophalangeal joints and digits as described previously. Large cystic lesion is identified within the calcaneus as previously seen.
2. Diffuse soft-tissue swelling and inferior calcaneal spur.

51. CT REPORT

CT of Abdomen

CLINICAL HISTORY: Increased liver enzyme.

TECHNIQUE: The patient was scanned from the dome of the diaphragm through the iliac crest after administration of oral and intravenous contrast.

COMPARISON: Comparison is made with a previous ultrasound examination dated 11/18/XX.

FINDINGS: Evaluation of the liver demonstrates mildly decreased attenuation to be present throughout the liver diffusely. No focal abnormalities are present within the liver. The spleen, pancreas, kidneys, and adrenal glands appear unremarkable. No enlarged lymph nodes are seen within the abdomen. No abnormal fluid collections are seen within the abdomen. The lung bases appear clear. No pleural effusions are seen.

IMPRESSION:

1. There is diffusely decreased attenuation present within the liver. This suggests the presence of fatty infiltration of the liver. No focal abnormalities are seen within the liver.
2. The remainder of the CT examination of the abdomen appears unremarkable.

52. LUNG SCAN REPORT

EXAMINATION OF: Ventilation-perfusion lung scan.

CLINICAL SYMPTOMS: Shortness of breath.

VENTILATION-PERFUSION LUNG SCAN:

DOSE: 2.0 millicuries of technetium-99m DTPA via aerosol. 6.0 millicuries of technetium-99m MAA IV. Comparison is made with chest radiograph obtained at the same time.

There is inhomogeneity regarding ventilatory scan. This is seen bilaterally. There appears to be elevation of the right hemidiaphragm.

There is decreased perfusion and ventilation along the right posterior lung base. The patient is noted to have pulmonary opacities and pleural effusions on chest radiograph. Small area of decreased perfusion and ventilation noted along the posterior aspect of the left upper lobe. Overall findings indeterminate for pulmonary embolus.

IMPRESSION: Indeterminate probability for pulmonary embolus.

53. MRI REPORT

EXAMINATION OF: Myocardial perfusion imaging.

CLINICAL SYMPTOMS: Chest pain, shortness of breath.

MYOCARDIAL PERFUSION IMAGING: CARDIOLITE HEART IMAGING: SPECT left ventricular myocardial perfusion imaging study was performed in this patient. 29.5 millicuries of technetium-99m sestamibi was injected intravenously at peak stress. The patient had a maximal heart rate of 88%.

Evaluation of the qualitative image series shows the left ventricular myocardium to have a normal uptake of tracer. There is no evidence to suggest myocardial infarction or stress-induced ischemia.

IMPRESSION: Normal Cardiolite heart imaging as described above.

54. FROM OPERATIVE REPORT 20

CLINICAL HISTORY: C/C clear cell CA pelvis.

SPECIMEN RECEIVED: A. Endocervical curettings. B. Endometrial biopsy.

GROSS DESCRIPTION:

A. The specimen is labeled with the patient's name and "ecc" and consists of specimen jar with negligible tissue. The specimen is filtered and placed in one cassette.
B. The specimen is labeled with the patient's name and "endometrial" and consists of approximately 1 cc of wispy fragments.

MICROSCOPIC DESCRIPTION:

A. Sections show no tissue after processing.

Sections show fragments of tissue consisting predominantly of endocervical tissue and lower uterine segment. The endometrial glands are lined by 1 to 2 layers of columnar epithelium. Malignant clear cell carcinoma is microscopically identified.

DIAGNOSIS:

A. Endocervical curettings: Malignant clear cell carcinoma identified.

Endometrial biopsy: Scant fragments of endocervical mucosa and lower uterine segment; Grade 3, secondary, malignant endocervix and endometrium clear cell carcinoma, primary site unknown.

55. FROM OPERATIVE REPORT 37

CLINICAL HISTORY: Bladder cancer.

SPECIMEN RECEIVED: Random bladder biopsy.

GROSS DESCRIPTION: The specimen is labeled with "biopsy" and consists of 3 specimens processed in toto, and random bladder pink-tan tissue biopsies in 1 cassette.

MICROSCOPIC DESCRIPTION: Sections show fragments of bladder mucosa showing vascularization and congestion with mild lymphocytic, plasma cell infiltrates, and lymphoid aggregates. The urothelium varies from normal to moderate to severe dysplasia to carcinoma in situ with full-thickness cytologic atypia and occasional mitoses. One fragment shows grade 2 papillary transitional cell carcinoma. The underlying lamina propria shows reactive fibroblasts with scattered lymphocytic, plasma cell, and eosinophilic infiltrates with admixed multinucleated giant cells. No definitive stromal invasion is identified.

DIAGNOSIS: Random bladder biopsies: Moderate to severe urothelial dysplasia/transitional cell carcinoma in situ and noninvasive grade 2 *(of 3)* papillary transitional cell carcinoma.

56. FROM OPERATIVE REPORT 31

CLINICAL HISTORY: Adenoma.

SPECIMEN RECEIVED: Cecal ascending polyp.

GROSS DESCRIPTION: Received in a container labeled "cecal ascending polyp" are three fragments of tan tissue measuring 0.3 to 0.4 cm diameter. The specimen is totally submitted.

MICROSCOPIC DESCRIPTION: The cecum and ascending mucosal fragments show glands that vary in size and configuration and are lined by uniform epithelial cells. Hyperplasia of the glandular and surface epithelium are prominent with serrated architectures evident.

DIAGNOSIS: Cecum and ascending colon biopsies, mucosal (three): Hyperplastic polyps (three).

57. FROM OPERATIVE REPORT 43

CLINICAL HISTORY: Lumbar herniated disc.

TISSUE RECEIVED: Lumbar disc.

GROSS DESCRIPTIONS: Submitted in formalin, labeled with the patient's name and "lumbar disc" are several irregular fragments of pink-tan ragged tissue measuring approximately 2 × 1.5 × 0.5 cm in aggregate. Submitted in toto.

MICROSCOPIC DESCRIPTIONS: The slide shows several irregular fragments of fibrocartilaginous intervertebral disc material. There are no significant inflammatory infiltrates or evidence of neoplasm.

DIAGNOSIS: Intervertebral disc, lumbar region, discectomy: fragments of intervertebral disc.

58. PATHOLOGY REPORT

SPECIMEN RECEIVED: A. polyps, cecum/sigmoid—adenoma. B. Barrett's esophagus—rule out dysplasia.

GROSS DESCRIPTION: The specimens are received in two containers:

A. In the container labeled "colon biopsy and polyp" are four fragments of tan-pink tissue measuring 0.3 to 0.6 cm diameter. The specimen is totally submitted as "A."
B. In the container labeled "Barrett's esophagus biopsy" are six fragments of tan-gray tissue measuring 0.1 to 0.3 cm diameter. The specimen is totally submitted.

MICROSCOPIC DESCRIPTION:

A. The mucosal fragments of the cecum and sigmoid colon show polypoid architectures with adenomatous features within surface and glandular epithelial sites. The glands vary in size and configuration and are lined by enlarged, mildly pleomorphic cells with elongated hyperchromatic nuclei.
B. The esophageal biopsies demonstrate gastric cardia mucosa exhibiting intestinal metaplasia. The glands vary in size and configuration and have uniform elongated epithelial cells. Separation by a fibrous lamina propria is evident.

DIAGNOSIS:

A. Cecum and sigmoid colon biopsies, mucosal: Adenomatous polyp fragments.
B. Esophageal biopsy: Gastric cardia mucosa with intestinal metaplasia, consistent with Barrett's esophagus.

59. FROM OPERATIVE REPORT 14

SPECIMEN RECEIVED: Muscle biopsy, left deltoid.

INDICATION: Deltoid muscle pain and swelling.

GROSS DESCRIPTION: Received in a container labeled "muscle biopsy left deltoid" is a fragment of brown tissue measuring 0.7 × 0.5 × 0.5 cm. The specimen is totally submitted.

MICROSCOPIC DESCRIPTION: The skeletal muscle of the left deltoid shows normal morphology.

DIAGNOSIS: Muscle biopsy, left deltoid: No pathologic diagnosis.

60. FROM OPERATIVE REPORT 7

CLINICAL HISTORY: Mass of axillary fold.

SPECIMEN RECEIVED: Lipoma from axillary fold.

GROSS DESCRIPTION: The specimen is labeled with the patient's name and "lipoma from axillary fold, intramuscular," which consists of a loosely encapsulated yellow adipose tissue, 8 × 7.8 × 1.8 cm. Sectioning reveals homogeneous yellow adipose tissue throughout. Representative sections in 4 cassettes.

MICROSCOPIC DIAGNOSIS: Mature adipose tissue consistent with lipoma, axillary fold.

61. PATHOLOGY REPORT

CLINICAL DIAGNOSIS AND HISTORY: Cyst.

TISSUE(S) SUBMITTED: Lesion, back.

GROSS DESCRIPTION: Specimen is received in fixative and consists of a 3.3 × 2.5 × 2.2-cm thin-walled cyst containing charcoal, gray-black, friable material.

MICROSCOPIC DESCRIPTION: One microscopic slide examined.

DIAGNOSIS: Follicular cyst, infundibular type, skin of back.

62. FROM OPERATIVE REPORT 12

CLINICAL HISTORY: Left ischial ulcer.

SPECIMEN RECEIVED: Ischial tissue *(left)*.

GROSS DESCRIPTION: Received in a container labeled "left ischial tissue" is an irregularly shaped fragment of soft tissue with a small portion containing an ellipse of skin. The specimen measures 18 × 7.5 × 6 cm in greatest dimension. The skin ellipse measures 4.5 × 2.5 × 0.3 cm. A central opening measuring 2 cm in greatest dimension is present. The remainder of the tissue has a nodular solid tan-gray to brown appearance. On sectioning diffuse fibrosis extends through the area. Representative portions are submitted.

MICROSCOPIC DESCRIPTION: The soft tissue of the left ischial region demonstrates extensive diffuse fibrosis with mild infiltrates of mononuclear inflammatory cells. A significant portion of the soft tissue is covered with granular fibrin containing sheets of neutrophils that rest upon a granulation tissue base. The adjacent epidermis shows pseudoepitheliomatous hyperplasia and normal maturation pattern.

DIAGNOSIS: Skin and soft tissue of left ischial region, excision: Granulation tissue, extensive, with diffuse fibrosis and mild chronic inflammation. Ulcer with mild to moderate acute inflammation.

63. FROM OPERATIVE REPORT 39

CLINICAL HISTORY: Morbid obesity.

SPECIMEN RECEIVED: Liver biopsy.

GROSS DESCRIPTION: The specimen is labeled with the patient's name and "liver biopsy" and consists of a 2 cm needle core of greenish tissue.

MICROSCOPIC DESCRIPTION: Sections show liver showing mild fatty change. The portal triads are unremarkable.

DIAGNOSIS: Liver biopsy showing mild fatty change.

64. FROM OPERATIVE REPORT 6

CLINICAL DIAGNOSIS AND HISTORY: Cyst.

TISSUE(S) SUBMITTED: Scalp cyst.

GROSS DESCRIPTION: Specimen is received in fixative and consists of an ovoid, rubbery, gray-white, 2 × 1.3 cm diameter cyst with gray-white laminated, friable contents.

MICROSCOPIC DESCRIPTION: One microscopic slide examined.

DIAGNOSIS: Follicular cyst, isthmus-catagen type (pilar cyst), clinically scalp.

65. FROM OPERATIVE REPORT 19

CLINICAL HISTORY: Left upper lobe abscess—probably secondary aspiration, culture and pseudomonas.

SPECIMEN RECEIVED: Lung, left upper lobe.

GROSS DESCRIPTION: Received in a container labeled "left upper lobe of lung" is a lung upper lobe measuring 17 × 11 × 3.4 cm as a collapsed specimen. The lobe weighs 283 grams. All surfaces have a dull gray yellow exudate that extends over the pleura. The pleura has a wrinkled collapsed appearance. On sectioning the majority of the lung parenchyma is replaced by a necrotic collapsed cyst with a ragged gray-yellow wall. This completely encompasses the vast majority of lung parenchyma with only small portions persisting in the base of the upper lobe. Bronchus and vascular structures are identified and appear unremarkable. Multiple representative sections of lung parenchyma are submitted.

MICROSCOPIC DESCRIPTION: The left upper lobe tissue sections show an extensive area of coagulation necrosis and marked destruction of the pulmonary parenchyma. Sheets of neutrophils are present within fibrin and coagulation necrosis debris. The adjacent lung tissue shows collections of macrophages and inflammatory cells within alveoli. Abundant fibrin debris accompanies the inflammation. Prominent squamous metaplasia is present within the bronchial tree that persists. Extensive interstitial fibrosis within the adjacent lung parenchyma is also present.

DIAGNOSIS: Lung, left upper lobe, resection: Abscess, large, with severe acute inflammation and extensive necrosis. Interstitial fibrosis with chronic inflammation, adjacent lung tissue.

66. FROM OPERATIVE REPORT 21

CLINICAL HISTORY: Atelectasis lung.

GROSS DESCRIPTION: 20 ml of mucoid fluid received in one container.

SPECIMEN RECEIVED: Bronchial washing.

SPECIMEN ADEQUACY: Specimen satisfactory for cytologic evaluation.

DIAGNOSIS: Atypical cells, cannot rule out malignancy.

COMMENTS: Rare groups of mildly atypical squamous cells present, significance and origin unknown. Cytology correlated with accompanying histology specimen. Please see pathology report.

Report amended due to transcription error on original. Discussed with Dr. Green.

67. FROM OPERATIVE REPORT 23

CLINICAL HISTORY: Pleural effusion, unknown cause.

GROSS DESCRIPTIONS: Ten ml bloody fluid received in one syringe.

SPECIMEN RECEIVED: Pleural fluid.

SPECIMEN ADEQUACY: Specimen satisfactory for cytologic evaluation.

DIAGNOSIS: No cytologic evidence of malignancy.

COMMENTS: Specimen shows predominantly lymphocytes.

68. 2/1/XX FAMILY PRACTICE SERVICE, MARK ADAMS, MD

(REPORTS 68 TO 79 ARE FOR THE SAME PATIENT)

This 68-year-old female presents to the office today requesting a complete physical examination. She recently moved to our area and states that she would like to establish with a family practitioner. She has a history of coronary artery disease, status post coronary artery bypass × 3 in 1978. She has been doing well. Gravid 3, para 3, postmenopausal about 20 years. History is also significant for hypertension, controlled by diet. Otherwise no complaints.

PAST MEDICAL HISTORY: Remarkable for conditions stated above.

OPERATIONS:

1. Hysterectomy with bladder repair, 1973
2. Bilateral blepharoplasty
3. D&C × 4

ALLERGIES: None.

MEDICATIONS: Digoxin 0.25 mg, Lasix 40 mg p.o. q.d., estrogen.

TOBACCO: Does not smoke.

ALCOHOL: Occasional.

SOCIAL HISTORY: Homemaker, mother of three. Husband recently transferred to area from California.

FAMILY HISTORY: Mother deceased from heart disease. Father has had multiple strokes. Two brothers, one with polio. Three children, health good. One sister, died of breast cancer at age 35.

REVIEW OF SYMPTOMS: Denies nausea, vomiting, headaches, dysuria, incontinence, dyspnea. Occasional bouts of atrial fibrillation; always converts spontaneously.

HEENT: Wears glasses. Otherwise negative.

RESPIRATORY: Negative.

CARDIOVASCULAR: Negative except as discussed above.

GI/GU: Postmenopausal, on estrogen.

ENDOCRINE: No diabetes or thyroid problems.

MUSCULOSKELETAL: Some arthritis, both hands.

PSYCHIATRIC: Negative.

PHYSICAL EXAMINATION: Reveals a very pleasant elderly female in no distress.

VITALS: Blood pressure is 140/84 right arm sitting position, 150/90 left arm sitting position; pulse 90 and regular.

WEIGHT: 115 lb.

SKIN: No skin lesions are present.

NODES: No lymphadenopathy.

ENT: Negative.

CHEST: Clear to auscultation.

CARDIAC: Reveals a regular rhythm. I did not hear any murmurs or gallops.

BREAST EXAMINATION: Right side free from lumps or masses. Small lump noted in left breast on examination, which is painless, without discharge, without retraction.

ASSESSMENT AND PLAN:

1. History of coronary artery disease, status post coronary artery bypass. No complaints at present, no abnormal findings. Continue medications as previously prescribed.
2. Breast mass on examination. Suggest mammography. If positive, consultation will be requested from surgery.
3. Postmenopausal, continue on estrogen therapy.

69. 2/2/XX JACOB BOND, MD

Patient has bilateral diagnostic mammography that shows normal finding on the right but dense, suspicious area on the left. Suggestion by radiologist is further clinical study.

70. 2/5/XX JACOB BOND, MD

Patient is seen today in the clinic at the request of Dr. Adams for evaluation of suspicious lump in the left breast. Patient states that she does not practice self-breast examination and therefore was unaware of the existing lump. She does state, however, on reflection, that the left breast at times was painful. No nipple discharge or puckering has been noted. Patient states that she has a sister who died of breast cancer in her mid-thirties. No other family history for cancer was noted.

EXAMINATION: Both breasts seem to be symmetrical. No abnormal findings on first view, right breast examination benign. Left breast identifies small lump where calcifications were noted on mammography.

ASSESSMENT: Left breast mass.

PLAN: Although it is difficult to say that this is not a single cyst, I would recommend a breast biopsy at patient's earliest convenience to rule out any possible malignancy. Options to include conservative measures of waiting for further signs, repeat mammography, 6-month breast checks were discussed with patient as well as risks and benefits of biopsy and possible mastectomy if findings are positive. Patient wishes to discuss with her husband and will let me know what she decides.

Thank you for asking me to consult on the care of Mrs. Smith. My recommendations are as above. I will await her further decision if she wishes further care from a surgical standpoint.

71. 2/8/XX JACOB BOND, MD

Phone call from patient wishing to schedule left breast biopsy. Scheduled for 2/10/XX by Dr. Bond.

72. 2/10/XX JACOB BOND, MD (ADMISSION SERVICE)

This patient is a 68-year-old female with chief complaint of left breast mass, admitted for left breast biopsy. The patient has a history of hypertension, coronary artery disease, and coronary artery bypass × 3. She also has a history of hysterectomy and is on estrogen therapy. She was in her usual state of health until a physical examination in early February, which revealed a small mass in the left breast. Mammography reportedly confirmed presence of mass and calcifications. Right breast exhibited no abnormal findings. The patient had menarche at age 12 and has given birth to three children. The patient has a family history positive for one sister with breast carcinoma. Medical history: as stated above for hypertension and CAD.

PHYSICAL EXAMINATION: Reveals a well-developed, well-nourished female in no apparent distress. The vital signs are stable, afebrile. The HEENT examination is within normal limits. The neck is supple, and the trachea is midline. No masses or adenopathy are present. The lungs are clear to auscultation and percussion. The cardiovascular examination is within normal limits. The left breast exhibits the presence of a small mass. The right breast is within normal limits. The right axilla is normal without adenopathy. The left axilla reveals small, less than 1 cm nonfixed, no matted lymph nodes. The abdominal examination is within normal limits. The rectal examination is normal, with guaiac-negative stool present in the vault.

ASSESSMENT: Left breast mass, admitted for breast biopsy and possible mastectomy.

73. 2/10/XX JACOB BOND, MD

Excisional breast biopsy was performed using local anesthesia. Pathology report documented adenocarcinoma of left breast. Patient was taken to operating room, administered general anesthesia, and underwent surgery the same day for mastectomy.

74. 2/10/XX JACOB BOND, MD

PREOPERATIVE DIAGNOSIS: Carcinoma of the left breast.

POSTOPERATIVE DIAGNOSIS: Same.

PROCEDURE PERFORMED: Left total mastectomy and left axillary node dissection. *(This is a modified radical mastectomy.)*

HISTORY: Patient underwent left breast biopsy for suspicious lesion 2/10/XX. Pathology report returned with diagnosis of adenocarcinoma of breast. Patient and her family discussed the benefits of the proposed total mastectomy and the risks, including death. Patient gives her understanding and agrees to proceed with the proposed procedure.

PROCEDURE: With the patient in the supine position under good general endotracheal anesthesia, a folded towel was placed beneath her left scapula and her left arm abducted on a pillow. She was prepped thoroughly with Betadine; the extent of her mastectomy incision was marked with a marking pen. We went about half an inch superior and half an inch inferior to her most medial circum-mammary incision, and it was a transverse incision. The draping was completed with Minnesota Mining drape and sterile paper in the usual manner. The superior flap was raised first. Bleeders on the breast were clamped and bovied; small bleeders on the flap were clamped and tied with 3-0 silk. The superior flap was raised to the clavicle inferior to the rectus sheath, medially to the sternal border, and laterally to the latissimus dorsi. The breast was outlined with a bovie, and then the breast was removed medially and laterally. We were somewhat concerned about involving the pectoralis muscle here, but it did not, and we could not see any invasion to the pectoralis fascia. Perforators were clamped and oversewn with 2-0 silk figure-of-eights. Small bleeders on the pectoralis major were bovied. The breast was allowed to fall laterally. The clavipectoral fascia was taken down. There was an area of scar tissue on the superior lateral portion of the pectoralis major attached to the breast, and we thought this was in the area of the previous biopsy. We had to dissect this off sharply, and it did not appear to be a cancer. Then she had a lot of inflammatory tissue in the axilla, which was rather difficult to define, but we exposed the axillary vein, hemoclipped the small venous tributaries, and dissected the axilla down to the 7th rib, and then took the breast off the serratus by bovie; the lateral chest bleeders were clamped and tied with 3-0 silk. The axilla was inspected, and the long thoracic and thoracodorsal nerve was intact. We left the superior branch of the intercostal brachial. It was dry. The mastectomy site was lavaged out with a liter of sterile water. Small bleeders were bovied. Several bleeders on the flaps were clamped and tied with 3-0 silk. The chest tubes were placed in the axilla and over the pectoralis major and exited laterally inferiorly, and the flaps were brought together without any tension with pulley sutures of 2-0 silk; then the wound was closed with a running 4-0 Prolene vertical mattress suture, removing the pulley sutures as we went. Vaseline dressings and dry dressings were applied.

Estimated blood loss was 400 ml. She tolerated this well. The flaps seemed to be intact. The drains were sewn into place and dry dressings applied. She tolerated the procedure well and was returned to the recovery room in good condition.

75. 2/12/XX JOYCE HARKNESS, MD, CONSULTING PHYSICIAN

CHIEF COMPLAINT: Atrial fibrillation.

Patient is a 68-year-old female, status post left total mastectomy for carcinoma of left breast. She has been doing fairly well postoperatively until this morning when she awoke with complaints of fluttering in the chest. ECG shows periods of rapid atrial fibrillation, with conversion to sinus rhythm spontaneously.

Past history is positive for CAD and hypertension. Patient is status post coronary artery bypass × 3. No chest pain or anginal symptoms have been noted.

Cardiac examination at present shows regular rate and rhythm; no gallops or murmurs are noted.

ASSESSMENT: Atrial fibrillation, status post left total mastectomy.

RECOMMENDATION: Treat conservatively with Coumadin at present. Monitor closely for signs of rhythm not converting spontaneously. Consideration would then have to be given to converting medically. Electrocardioversion is not recommended at this time.

76. 2/14/XX ANTHONY CASH, MD, CONSULTING PHYSICIAN

CHIEF COMPLAINT: Second-opinion surgery consultation *(inpatient)* regarding acute onset of no palpable pulses in lower extremities.

Mrs. Smith is a 68-year-old female with known history of CAD, status post coronary bypass in the 1970s. She recently underwent a total mastectomy 2/10/XX by Dr. Bond. Postoperatively, the patient has had an unremarkable course. Diet and activity were gradually increased. This morning she got up from bed about 4:30 and was weighed and had no problems. About 6:30 she suddenly experienced an acute onset of bilateral leg pain. The pain was excruciating. She was lying in bed when this first occurred. The surgical service was consulted about 7:30 this morning. By history from the patient, the pain gradually decreased. At the time of initial examination, she was complaining of a greater pain in her left thigh. She did state that her right leg had more of a numb feeling. She claimed that both legs were heavy feeling and that she would have to move every now and then to get relief from the pain.

Pertinent history reveals that the patient has been intermittently in atrial fibrillation. She has received two doses of Coumadin postoperatively for this atrial fibrillation.

Initial examination of the patient reveals a well-developed, well-nourished white female in no apparent distress. Heart: Regular rate and rhythm. Lungs are clear to auscultation bilaterally. Chest: The patient has a well-healing incision. There are no signs of infection, such as erythema or discharge. Abdomen: Positive bowel sounds, soft, nontender, nondistended. No rigidity on palpation. Examination of the pulses reveals the following: 2/4 in the radial, 2/4 in the carotid. No palpable pulses from the femoral on down. The patient does have Dopplerable pulses in the femorals bilaterally. She has Dopplerable left posterior tibial and no Dopplerable right dorsalis pedis pulse. Neuro: Cranial nerves II–XII grossly intact.

IMPRESSION: Probable saddle embolus to the distal aorta.

PLAN: Patient in need of emergent embolectomy with possible aortofemoral reconstruction. Acute onset of bilateral leg pain and numbness. Embolism most likely from left atrium. Patient has been in and out of atrial fibrillation postoperatively. Discussed the risks, benefits, and complications of the procedure with the patient. The patient understands she will be cared for postoperatively in the surgical intensive care unit.

Thank you for this interesting consultation. We agree with your initial assessment and are happy to participate in the care of this nice lady.

77. 2/14/XX JACOB BOND, MD

PREOPERATIVE DIAGNOSIS: Saddle embolus, distal aorta.

POSTOPERATIVE DIAGNOSIS: Same.

PROCEDURE PERFORMED: Bilateral aortofemoral embolectomy via femoral artery approach, femoral embolectomy.

PROCEDURE: The patient was placed in the supine position and given a general anesthetic. She was prepped from her nipples to her toes. Following this, two bilateral groin incisions were made and dissection was carried down. The common femoral, profunda femoral, and superficial femoral arteries were identified on both sides and controlled with vessel loops. Following this, starting with the right side, a linear arteriotomy was made over the superficial femoral artery and profunda arteries. No. 3 Fogarty catheters were passed distally down the superficial femoral arteries and profunda arteries. No thrombus was recovered. They were then flushed with heparinized saline and controlled with vessel loops. Following this, no. 4 and no. 6 Fogarty catheters were sequentially placed up the common femoral artery toward the iliofemoral area. A lot of thrombus was removed, and good arterial inflow was established in the right leg. Before any arteriotomies had been made, the patient had been given 5000 units of IV heparin that had been given 5 minutes to circulate.

Following this, the arteriotomy on the right was closed with a running 5-0 Prolene suture. Before the arteriotomy was closed, it was back-flushed and fore-flushed. The clamps and vessel loops were all removed, and flow was restored to the right lower extremity. The patient had Dopplerable posterior tibial pulses and palpable dorsalis pedis pulses at this point. Following this, a similar incision was made in the left lower extremity, and catheters were placed distally down the profunda and superficial femoral arteries, also flushing them sequentially with heparinized saline. No thrombus was removed from the distal arteries on the left; following this, no. 4 and no. 6 Fogarty catheters were placed sequentially toward the iliofemoral artery and more thrombotic material was removed, restoring good arterial inflow. The arteriotomy on the left was closed in a similar fashion with running 5-0 Prolene. All the clamps were removed. There were palpable dorsalis pedis and Dopplerable posterior tibial pulses at this junction of the procedure. Following this, both wounds were irrigated free of clot and debris. They were closed with three layers of interrupted 3-0 Vicryl, and the skin was closed with staples. The patient tolerated the procedure well and went to the recovery room in good condition.

78. 2/17/XX ERIC ARNOLD, MD, CONSULTING PHYSICIAN

REASON FOR CONSULTATION: Pleural effusion.

Patient is a 68-year-old female who was initially admitted for a left breast biopsy. Pathology confirmed carcinoma, and patient proceeded to have left total mastectomy. Hospital course has been complicated by atrial fibrillation and saddle embolism, requiring embolectomy. Patient is now 4 days postop embolectomy and has developed persistent pleural effusion. Attempts at medical management have failed, and patient is developing respiratory failure. A pleuracentesis is accomplished, with 500 ml of blood-tinged fluid immediately aspirated. Patient appears to receive immediate relief. Patient will be closely monitored in intensive care unit for additional signs of respiratory failure.

79. 3/10/XX JACOB BOND, MD

Patient in for follow-up appointment, as status post mastectomy on 2/10/XX. Hospital course was complicated by atrial fibrillation and embolism, requiring embolectomy. Patient also developed pleural effusion requiring pleuracentesis. Patient has now been discharged from the hospital for 10 days. Other than some incisional pain, patient seems to be doing well. No major complaints: denies shortness of breath, nausea, loss of appetite, fever, or pain in extremities. Energy levels seem to be returning to normal. Incision sites are examined, with no erythema or infection noted. Sutures are removed. Patient is instructed not to lift, push, or pull objects and to return to activities slowly. Wound care is reviewed. Patient is instructed to follow-up in 2 weeks or sooner if complaints.

80. PULMONARY FUNCTION STUDY

This 49-year-old presents with dyspnea. He has previous cigarette smoking history.

COMPLETE PULMONARY FUNCTION STUDY: Forced vital capacity is 4.87 L, 112% of predicted. FEV1 is 4.02 L, 113% of predicted. FEV1 is 83%. FEF 25% to 75% is normal. There is no significant response to bronchodilators. Flow volume loop shows a well-preserved inspiratory limb.

Total lung capacity by plethysmography is 6.82 L, 111% predicted. RV/TLC ratio and airway resistance are normal. Corrected DLCO was 18.99, 70% of predicted.

IMPRESSION:

1. Normal expiratory flow rates.
2. Normal lung volumes.
3. Mild reduction of DLCO is noted.

The cause of decreased diffusion capacity is unclear in this patient. Possible causes could include heart disease, pulmonary embolism, anemia, obstructive sleep apnea. Clinical correlation is advised for cause of abnormal diffusion. There is no evidence of coexisting obstructive or restrictive pulmonary disease.

Note: The items to be coded listed below:

- Spirometry before and after bronchodilator
- Respiratory flow volume loop
- Functional residual capacity

- Carbon monoxide diffusing capacity
- Bronchodilator supply

81. OPERATIVE REPORT

PREOPERATIVE DIAGNOSIS: History of adenocarcinoma of the prostate.

POSTOPERATIVE DIAGNOSIS: History of adenocarcinoma of the prostate.

PROCEDURES PERFORMED:

1. Transrectal ultrasound performance with:
   a. Volume study.
   b. Needle localization.
   c. Needle implantation.
   d. Cystoscopy.

ANESTHESIA: General.

ESTIMATED BLOOD LOSS: Minimal.

PROCEDURE: Please see the preoperative note for indications of the procedure, as well as full informed consent. The patient underwent a general anesthetic and was put in the extended dorsal lithotomy position. The table was decanted or in Trendelenburg 5 degrees. He was prepped and draped in the usual fashion, which included a 14-French Foley catheter with 120 ml of sterile saline in his bladder. The testicles and scrotum had been taped back and away. We irrigated the rectum with sterile saline, performing a pseudo-enema. The patient underwent transrectal ultrasound placement. This was connected to the gantry. The placement of ultrasound and the grid work were set up so that the base of the prostate is noted at #1 on the grid work. The anterior most component at approximately 4.5–5, prostate extended from side-to-side from A to F.

Five-mm increment imaging slices were obtained, starting at the base of the prostate, carrying it back for a total of 3 cm to 30. Volume of the prostate is approximately 33 ml.

The outline of the prostate was drawn during the volume study. This information was given to the computer electronically so that a plan could be developed. Once the plan had been completed, the placement of the needles was performed in the usual fashion. The dose was delivered via 125 seeds after placement of the needles.

The total number of needles was 41 for 107 seeds (radioelements) placed with ultrasound guidance. The patient tolerated this well. At the conclusion, the patient was re-prepped and draped with the Foley catheter being removed and a cystoscopic evaluation was performed. There is no evidence of perforation of the urethra, bladder neck, or bladder. Urine within the bladder was clear. No seeds or spacers could be identified. An 18-French Foley catheter was then placed along with Triple antibiotic salve to the perineum and mesh panties. He tolerated the procedure well overall. Estimated blood loss minimal.

82. OPERATIVE REPORT

PREOPERATIVE DIAGNOSIS: History of a nodular mass, mid-prostate with urinary retention.

POSTOPERATIVE DIAGNOSIS: History of a nodular mass, mid-prostate with urinary retention; possible macronodular prostate.

PROCEDURE: Cystoscopy, transurethral resection of the prostate, one stage.

ANESTHESIA: Spinal.

ESTIMATED BLOOD LOSS: Approximately 100 ml.

FINDINGS: Benign prostatic hypertrophy type changes.

This is a 76-year-old gentleman who has a history as outlined in the preoperative note. Cystoscopically there is a large, red, macronodular area along the base of the prostate, which has been noted. The patient is having outlet obstructing symptoms. He has some decompensation in his urinary bladder but in discussion with the findings he wishes to go through the transurethral resection of prostate as outlined and discussed.

The patient underwent a spinal anesthetic, was put in the dorsolithotomy position, prepped, and draped in the usual fashion. Cystoscopic evaluation reveals the 1-cm nodule along the base of the prostate. This appears more macronodular but is not really prostatic or is very minimally prostatic. It could represent a deteriorating median lobe.

Resection of the prostate was started at the 12-o'clock position and was carried between 3 and 9 o'clock back to the plane of the verumontanum. The base tissue and the rest of the lateral walls were then resected. This was a pretty small prostate, around 20 ml of tissue. The area was separately resected.

At the conclusion of this procedure, the chips were irrigated out of the bladder. Final hemostasis was achieved. A 22-French three-way Foley catheter was inserted, inflated, and irrigated with slightly tinged irrigant returning. He was taken to the Recovery Room in satisfactory condition.

83. OPERATIVE REPORT

PREOPERATIVE DIAGNOSIS: History of left cryptorchid testicle.

POSTOPERATIVE DIAGNOSIS: Left ectopic testicle.

PROCEDURE PERFORMED: Left groin exploration with orchiopexy.

ANESTHESIA: General.

Please see the preoperative note for indications of the procedure as well as full informed consent. This 14-year-old was recognized on a sports physical as having a nonpalpable testicle. Through his younger years, it had been palpable.

The testicle on physical exam sat in the superficial inguinal canal next to the external ring. With him asleep, we went ahead and evaluated again and, again, the testicular cord was foreshortened, not allowing the testicle to get into the scrotum proper and sat slightly lateral as noted on the preoperative note.

He underwent a general anesthetic as noted previously and was prepped and draped in the usual fashion. A transverse incision was made halfway between the anterosuperior iliac spine and pubic tubercle at the presumed location of the internal ring. The external oblique aponeurosis was opened along the course of its fibers to the external ring. The inguinal canal was opened. The external ilioinguinal nerve was identified and preserved. The testicle could be identified outside the inguinal canal lateral to it in its own small covering. This was opened and the cord, with the testicle, could be freed up. We removed some of the adhesions along the cord, which allowed very satisfactory length to allow it to fit well into the inferior aspect of the left hemiscrotum.

A separate incision was made in the left hemiscrotum. Subdartos pouch was formed using sharp and blunt dissection. The testicle was brought through in a medial tract performed by using blunt dissection with a hemostat. The testicle was brought down into the scrotum and out of the incision with ease. On the inferior pole of the testicle, a small 3-0 chromic was placed in the inferior most portion of the septum. The scrotal wall was then closed over the testicle with interrupted 3-0 chromic. Irrigation of the wound was performed. No active bleeding could be identified. The external oblique aponeurosis was closed utilizing 3-0 silk. Bupivacaine 0.25% without epinephrine was placed approximately 3 ml in the internal ring and 3 ml in the subcut. The subcut was closed with interrupted 3-0 chromic and 4-0 undyed Vicryl for subcuticular incision closure with Steri-Strips. He tolerated the procedure well.

84. TRANSURETHRAL NEEDLE ABLATION (TUNA) THERAPY

The procedure was performed in the usual fashion and multiple segments as noted.

Transrectal ultrasound was performed with the patient in the left lateral position. The ultrasound is performed in order to evaluate the prostate in detail, bladder neck, and seminal vesicles. Ultrasound shows a width of the prostate at 45 mm. The entire calculated volume of the prostate is approximately 40 cc's. Large amount of the bladder neck/median lobe is noted as prominent. No other findings are noted in the prostate.

A prostatic block was then performed. Using an 83, 18-gauge spinal needle, the area between the "angle" of the prostate to seminal vesicle laterally is identified. Needle is placed into position at that point under the rectum. 8 cc's of 2% Xylocaine are used to create the block.

The patient was then brought to the cystoscopic area. Further preparation includes viscous Xylocaine and liquid Xylocaine to the bladder. After a 15-minute wait, we proceeded with the procedure as follows.

The scope was advanced down into the urethra through the sphincter and prostatic urethra and into the bladder. A prominent bladder neck is noted. The length of the prostate is about 28 mm. The obstructing components are definitely the median lobe.

After introduction of the radiofrequency thermotherapy stylet, treatments were performed utilizing a suggested needle-length of 16 mm.

The treatments were performed 1 cm back from the bladder neck laterally. One cm back from that positioning, the next treatment halfway between the original and the verumontanum. This was performed bilaterally. All target temperatures were reached without difficulty. The fifth treatment zone was the median lobe. We retracted the needles to 12 mm to do this. The patient tolerated the procedure well. Foley catheter was placed at the conclusion of the procedure. Usual post procedure protocol to include antibiotics and pain relief medications.

85. OPERATIVE REPORT

PREOPERATIVE DIAGNOSIS: Glaucoma, severe stage, open angle, right eye.

POSTOPERATIVE DIAGNOSIS: Same.

OPERATION PERFORMED: Sequential cyclocryotherapy, right eye.

INDICATION: This 74-year-old white female has an out-of-control glaucoma in her right eye. She is pseudophakic and has been allergic to multiple drops and has had one sequential therapy before that worked quite well and then she stopped taking her drops. It is obvious that despite the cyclocryotherapy, she will need to continue on the Pilocarpine.

DESCRIPTION OF PROCEDURE: After the patient was placed on the OR table, she was given a retrobulbar anesthesia of Xylocaine 2% with 0.75% Marcaine and Wydase for a volume of 3.5 cc. After this, she was prepped and draped in the usual sterile fashion for ophthalmic surgery and a wire lid speculum was used to separate the lids of the right eye. 3.5 mm from the limbus was marked out with a marking pen in the superior temporal quadrant and the right inferior nasal quadrant of her eye. The cryoprobe was liquid nitrogen and nitrous oxide and was applied to –80 for a 5-second treatment in a freeze-thaw-freeze triple row of cryotherapy laid down in both the defined quadrants. There were no complications. Maxitrol ointment, Telfa, and two pads were applied and the patient sent to the Recovery Room.

86. OPERATIVE REPORT

PREOPERATIVE DIAGNOSES:

1. Blunt trauma with paint ball, right eye.
2. Hyphema, right eye, secondary to #1.
3. Recurrent hyphema, right eye, secondary to #1.
4. Corneal staining, right eye, secondary to #1.
5. Increased intraocular pressure, right eye, secondary to #l.
6. Dense cataract, right eye, secondary to #1.

POSTOPERATIVE DIAGNOSIS: Same.

PROCEDURE PERFORMED: Irrigation and aspiration of hyphema and blood clot anterior chamber, right eye.

ANESTHESIA: General endotracheal anesthesia.

INDICATION: This 14-year-old white male has had persistent problems since he was hit with a paint ball in his right eye 2 weeks ago. It has not resolved. It has continued to bleed and now it has formed a huge clot. Because of the increase in pain and obvious corneal staining, it was elected to irrigate the clot at this time. No guarantees were made to the mother for vision.

DESCRIPTION OF PROCEDURE: After the patient was prepped and draped in the usual sterile fashion for ophthalmic surgery under general endotracheal anesthesia, a wire lid speculum was used to separate the lids of the right eye. The Super knife was then used in the limbal area to make a 2-mm–wide incision at the 8-o'clock meridian, and the chamber was filled with BSS Plus. Using the Simcoe I&A apparatus, gentle suction, and a push-pull method, the clot was removed and the blood was irrigated. There was no damage done to the lens surface or to the iris and the pupil remained round. Healon was used to help dissolve the clot and make it easier for aspiration. At the end of the procedure, all the Healon and blood clot was removed and the pupil remained round. There was a dense cataract well on its way to hypermaturity already present, but no evidence of any vitreous or subluxation of the lens. The wound was closed with a 10-0 nylon suture, and the knot was buried. Healon was then placed over the cornea because the cornea showed some irregularity secondary to the paint ball explosion. Solu-Medrol was injected inferiorly Sub-Tenon's. Atropine 1% was placed in the eye and Maxitrol ointment and a Telfa pad, patch, and shield applied. The patient was sent to the Recovery Room. There were no complications.

87. OPERATIVE REPORT

PREOPERATIVE DIAGNOSES:

1. Cataract, right eye.
2. Pseudophakia, left eye.
3. Excess myopia, both eyes.
4. Diabetes mellitus.
5. Atrial fibrillation, controlled.
6. Hypothyroidism.
7. Pacemaker for history of bradycardia.

POSTOPERATIVE DIAGNOSIS: Same.

PROCEDURE PERFORMED: Extracapsular cataract extraction, right eye, with insertion of intraocular lens implant, right eye.

ANESTHESIA: MAC anesthesia.

INDICATION: This 86-year-old white female has had progressively decreasing vision in her right eye secondary to a nuclear sclerotic cataract that has reduced her vision to 20/400, which can be corrected to 20/100. She had successful cataract surgery in her left eye a year ago and has returned to 20/40 vision without glasses. She was counseled again as to the type of procedure, the need for medical clearance, anticoagulation regulation, and pacemaker regulation.

PROCEDURE: After the patient was placed on the OR table, she was given Nadbath and Van Lint anesthesia on a 25-gauge needle for a volume of 9 cc of Xylocaine 2% with 0.75% Marcaine and Wydase. The same mixture was administered on a blunt retrobulbar Atkinson needle for a volume of 4 cc without complications. After this, she was prepped and draped in the usual sterile fashion for ophthalmic surgery, and the Honan balloon was placed for 4 minutes by the clock at 35 mm Mercury. After this, the lid speculum was used to separate the lids of the right eye and a fornix-based flap was raised from 9 o'clock to 3 o'clock and the wet-field cautery was used. There was no excessive bleeding despite the use of the Coumadin. A 69-Beaver blade made a half-thickness O'Malley groove from 9:30 to 2:30 and the Super knife was used to enter the eye at 11 o'clock. The chamber was filled with Healon, and a dry, nonirrigating anterior capsulotomy was performed on a bent 25-gauge needle. The wound was extended with left and right corneal-cutting scissors, and three 8-0 Vicryls were post placed. Using a lens vectis, the nucleus was expressed without capsular rupture or iris prolapse. The post placed sutures were tied down and the Simcoe I&A apparatus was used to clean up excess cortex. It was noted that there was very weak zonular support and positive vitreous pressure. We elected at this point to fill the chamber with Healon, insert a lens glide, and a 14 diopter L122 UV lens was inserted. Miochol was used to bring down the pupil and eight 10-0 nylons were used to close the wound. A peripheral iridectomy was performed at 1 o'clock and there was no evidence of any vitreous. The Healon was left in the eye. The pupil was round and two 8-0 Vicryls closed the conjunctiva. Solu-Medrol was used sub-Tenon's inferiorly, and Pilopine gel, Maxitrol ointment, Telfa, two pads, and an eye shield were applied. There were no complications, and the heart rate was not out of ordinary since it was protected with a magnet.

88. OPERATIVE REPORT

PREOPERATIVE DIAGNOSES:

1. History of corneoscleral laceration, right eye.
2. History of retained sutures, right eye.

POSTOPERATIVE DIAGNOSIS: Same.

PROCEDURE PERFORMED: Removal of retained sutures, anterior cornea, right eye.

ANESTHESIA: General anesthesia.

INDICATIONS: This 17-year-old white male who suffered a severe injury to his eye with multiple lacerations of his right cornea has now recovered to the point that his vision is correctable with a contact lens to 20/25; however, there is a large amount of suture material, and it was elected to remove the sutures at this time.

PROCEDURE: After the patient was prepped and draped in the usual sterile fashion for ophthalmic surgery and he was under general anesthesia, the lid speculum was used to separate the lids of the right eye. Healon was placed over the sutures, a Super knife was used to cut them, and they were pulled with a combination of straight tiers and 0.12 forceps. One suture remained deeply buried and was left alone. None of the scleral sutures were removed. There were no complications and the chamber remained intact. He was patched with TobraDex ointment without Telfa for 24 hours, and we will make arrangements to see him within the week.

89. OPERATIVE REPORT

PREOPERATIVE DIAGNOSIS: Splenic hematoma.

POSTOPERATIVE DIAGNOSIS: Same.

PROCEDURE PERFORMED: Splenectomy.

ANESTHESIA: General.

PROCEDURE: A surgical technique was used to remove the spleen due to splenic hematoma following trauma in a football game, kicked. The patient was given general anesthesia. The anesthesiologist inserted a temporary tube into the patient's stomach to empty it. This helped to decompress the stomach and prevent postoperative nausea. A catheter was inserted into the bladder to drain the urine. Surgery was done with the patient lying flat on his back. Several small incisions were made into the abdomen. One was used for the laparoscope, which was attached to a camera that sent images to the video monitor. The other incisions were used to hold or manipulate tissue in the abdomen. Carbon dioxide gas is insufflated into the abdominal cavity to allow room to work and to allow visualizing the area. Parts of the spleen were freed from surrounding tissue. Blood vessels to the stomach and spleen were visualized, clipped with metal clips, and divided. Once the spleen was dissected free of its attachments in the abdominal cavity, it was placed in a special surgical plastic bag and removed through one of the small abdominal incisions. At the end of the surgery, carbon dioxide gas was removed. The small incisions were closed with suture, the skin cleaned, and the incisions covered with a small dressing. Patient tolerated the procedure well.

90. RECORD OF OPERATION

PREOPERATIVE DIAGNOSIS: Prostate cancer.

POSTOPERATIVE DIAGNOSIS: Same.

PROCEDURE PERFORMED: Cryoablation of prostate including suprapubic catheter insertion, transrectal ultrasound for prostate volume determination, placement of probes, and guidance of tissue ablation. Suprapubic catheter insertion.

CLINICAL NOTE: This gentleman has had prostate cancer. He has elected to proceed with cryoablation.

PROCEDURE NOTE: The patient was given a spinal anesthetic, prepped and draped in the lithotomy position. The Foley catheter placed into the bladder and transrectal ultrasound probe introduced. Prostate measurements and volumes were determined. Using the Cryoguide system, an 8 probe freeze was selected. Probes were placed under ultrasound guidance. Once all temperature monitors and Cryoprobes were placed, the Foley catheter was withdrawn and patient then cystoscoped using the flexible instrument. This ensured the needles had not violated the urethra and the probes were in good position. A 12-French suprapubic catheter was then placed using a trocar technique under endoscopic and ultrasound guidance into the anterior wall of the bladder using a single pass technique. Once probe position was confirmed the urethral warming catheter was placed over a guide wire. A two cycle freeze was undertaken; please see the details. Temperature was recorded in the operative part of the chart. Ice bulb was monitored on ultrasound guidance. At the end of the procedure Cryoprobe was withdrawn. A Foley catheter was placed because of hematuria. CBI was started. Five minutes of pressure was applied to the perineum. Bacitracin ointment was applied to the perineum. The patient tolerated the procedure well and was transferred to the recovery room in good condition.

91. CLINIC PROCEDURE

PREOPERATIVE DIAGNOSIS: Left shoulder bursitis.

POSTOPERATIVE DIAGNOSIS: Same.

PROCEDURE PERFORMED: Left shoulder injection.

PROCEDURE: After obtaining consent, the patient was brought to the Special Procedures area. His left shoulder area was cleaned with Betadine. 7 cc of lidocaine and 1 cc of Kenalog were injected in his left subacromial bursa without complications. The patient was slightly nauseated. His blood pressure was 168/107. Heart rate was 79/minute and regular.

I was planning on injecting his right shoulder; however, because of his symptoms I elected to withhold that at this time and do it at some other time.

92. REPORT OF OPERATION

PREOPERATIVE DIAGNOSIS: Left renal calculus.

POSTOPERATIVE DIAGNOSIS: Same.

PROCEDURE PERFORMED: Left ESWL *(extracorporeal shock wave lithotripsy)*.

CLINICAL NOTE: This gentleman came in with renal colic; a stent was placed. He presents now for ESWL. The patient was given a general laryngeal mask anesthetic, prepped, and draped in the supine position. Stone targeted and shock head engaged. A total of 2400 shocks at maximum KV and stone partial fragmentation and dissolution could be seen. The patient tolerated the procedure well and transferred to the recovery room in good condition. He will be seen in follow-up in 2 weeks' time for KUB.

93. REPORT OF OPERATION

PREOPERATIVE DIAGNOSIS: Acute renal failure, possible rejection, possible ischemic nephropathy.

POSTOPERATIVE DIAGNOSIS: Same.

PROCEDURE PERFORMED: Transplant kidney biopsy.

PROCEDURE: The transplant kidney in the right iliac fossa was visualized with ultrasound. The previous arteriovenous malformation was noted in the lower pole. We avoided that area as much as we could. At least three core biopsies were obtained after prepping the area in the usual fashion and injecting 1% lidocaine. A post biopsy ultrasound showed no evidence of hematoma or new AVN. The patient had some pain after the procedure and was sent to the procedure area. She will be getting some intravenous morphine.

Hemoglobin will be done in 6 hours.

94. WALKING OXYGEN DESATURATION STUDY

ENTRANCE DIAGNOSIS: Dyspnea. He gave a board rating of 5 by the time he finished; it was 3 at the beginning and showed some discomfort or effort to do this. He was able to walk 6 minutes at a slow pace without stopping. He did have some wheezing, some coughing, and was able to go 300 feet, which for this age group is relatively poor exercise tolerance. The 02 sats never dropped below 92%.

This patient does not need oxygen therapy with this form of exercise.

95. CLINIC PROGRESS NOTE

SUBJECTIVE: This is a 42-year-old Caucasian female who presents to the clinic today to establish with me as her primary care provider. At this particular visit she is complaining of right hip pain. She also complains of a nagging dry cough and would like to find out what might possibly be causing that. Her right hip pain has been going on for about 3 months now, which is constant and is aggravated by standing up from sitting. She does not feel the pain as much when walking and she says that this pain sometimes radiates to the buttocks and all the way down to her heel area. She occasionally feels a tingling sensation at the lateral aspect of the thigh, particularly at night. She has been treating this with over-the-counter pain medication but that is not found to be helpful. In terms of her cough, she noticed that she usually gets this whenever she has heartburn.

PAST MEDICAL HISTORY is remarkable for:

1. Gastroesophageal reflux disease and has been taking medication for this but she cannot recall the name of that medication right now.

2. She also was found to have only one kidney and this was thought to be congenital.
3. Obesity.

PAST SURGICAL HISTORY is remarkable for a hysterectomy due to a bicornuate uterus.

SCREENINGS: She gets a Pap smear and mammogram every year. Last time was last year, which were normal.

ALLERGIES: She otherwise has no known drug allergies.

FAMILY MEDICAL HISTORY: Her father died at the age of 70 from a myocardial infarction. Mother is presently having high blood pressure and is taking medication for her heart. She also has high blood cholesterol. She is presently 67 years old. There is one brother who has spondylitis, and she has a total of three other sisters. One sister has a benign breast tumor.

PERSONAL AND SOCIAL HISTORY: She is married. She has been doing this job for about 11 years now. She denies alcohol use. She has a total of two children. One is 18 years old and one is 6 years old. She had a miscarriage and one stillbirth.

REVIEW OF SYSTEMS: Constitutional: Head and neck, chest and lungs, cardiovascular, gastrointestinal, genitourinary, and extremities are otherwise negative other than what is already mentioned above.

OBJECTIVE FINDINGS: Vital signs: Blood pressure is 110/70. Pulse rate of 88. Weight is 202 pounds. General survey: She is an obese middle-aged lady who is pleasant in no acute distress. Head and neck: Normocephalic and atraumatic. Pink conjunctivae. Pupils are equal, round, and reactive to light and accommodation. Extraocular movements are intact. Neck is supple. No jugular venous distention. No carotid bruit. No thyromegaly. No cervical lymphadenopathy. Chest and lungs: Symmetrical expansion. Clear breath sounds. No roles or wheezes. Cardiovascular: Normal rate and regular rhythm. No murmur and no gallop. Abdomen is obese, soft; normoactive bowel sounds; nontender. No organomegaly. Extremities: She has no edema, cyanosis, or clubbing. Palpable distal pulses. Straight-leg testing on both lower extremities is essentially negative. She has pain on internal rotation of the right hip joint. No pain on external rotation. On the left side internal and external rotation of the hip joints are negative.

ASSESSMENT/PLAN:

1. Hip pain, exact etiology is uncertain but this could be most likely secondary to degenerative joint disease of the hip versus mild trochanteric bursitis. Superficial femoral nerve syndrome is also a consideration but not very likely. Discussed management with patient and we will just continue to observe for now. I advised her to give us a call when she develops progression of symptoms and referral to Orthopedics might be appropriate if that happens.
2. Cough, dry, probably related to heartburn symptoms.

96. TRANSESOPHAGEAL ECHOCARDIOGRAM REPORT

INDICATIONS: Evaluation of the aortic valve considering the stenosis that was not well documented angiographically.

PROCEDURE: The patient received 2 mg of Versed, and a transesophageal probe was advanced to the lower part of the esophagus. We had good visualization of the heart. The mitral valve was thickened with slight prolapse, but there was no significant regurgitation noted. The LV displayed normal size and normal function. The aortic root is normal in size. The aortic valve is calcified with diffuse cusp excursions with still adequate opening. Valve area was variable in different incidents varying from 1 to even above 2.

CONCLUSION: This transesophageal echo shows aortic valve disease but does not appear to be severe. It appeared to be moderately stenotic, and considering the angiography and the hemodynamics, this patient does not need valve surgery yet.

97. OPERATIVE REPORT

PREOPERATIVE DIAGNOSIS:

1. Steal syndrome, left hand.
2. Ischemic/necrotic ulcer of the left fifth digit.
3. End-stage renal disease.

POSTOPERATIVE DIAGNOSIS:

1. Steal syndrome, left hand.
2. Ischemic/necrotic ulcer of the left fifth digit.
3. End-stage renal disease.

PROCEDURE PERFORMED: Takedown of left arteriovenous fistula.

ANESTHESIA: IV Sedation

INDICATION: Andrea is a 55-year-old female who has end-stage renal disease and is on hemodialysis. She has had a fistula placed in her left arm. This is coming off either the radial, ulnar, or brachial artery and going to the cephalic vein. This is not functioning any longer. The remainder of the cephalic vein and venous system is not dilated. However, it is functional, as you can feel that there is a good thrill present. Some of this is going into a deeper venous system. However, in the interim she has developed ischemic pain in her left hand. Also, she has a wound on the tip of her left fifth digit that is not healing. She had accidentally cut it with a knife a while ago. It is not healing and is slowly getting worse. She currently is being dialyzed through a port system. She has even had problems with this and has had to undergo revision for this. She is not using the AVF in her arm, as this is not functional as far as being able to do dialysis. She also underwent Doppler studies of it this morning. With the graft open, she has no flow out to fingertips. With the fistula occluded by handheld pressure, her pressures are running up to the 30s. We discussed the procedure of a takedown of this fistula. We discussed the risk of bleeding, infection, and nerve injury and the significance of this. We also met with her in the Holding area again this morning preoperatively. She had no new questions. She understands and wishes to proceed with takedown of the left arm arteriovenous fistula.

PROCEDURE: The patient was brought to the operating room and placed in the supine position. After receiving IV sedation, she was prepped and draped in a sterile fashion. A transverse incision line 1 fingerbreadth below the antecubital fossa was marked out and infiltrated with 0.5% Marcaine. This was on the left arm. After waiting a couple of minutes, an incision was made. Dissection was carried down through the subcutaneous tissues. The venous limb of the arteriovenous fistula was identified. This was dissected out and controlled with vessel loops. We dissected out a segment so we would be able to transect this and ligate it. We then identified the artery. We did not dissect this out completely or circumferentially. We dissected out to identify where it was to be sure that we had two separate vascular structures and what we were going to be dividing was the venous limb and not the arterial limb. We checked Doppler flow in the hand and in the fingertips when we occluded the graft. We could then get flow in the digital arteries, as well as greatly augment the Doppler signal in the palmar arch and even in the radial and ulnar vessels. When we occluded the artery, we lost signals in the hand. Therefore we identified for sure our fistula. Again, by taking this down, we were going to increase the flow into the hand and especially into the fingertips. We then oversewed each end with a 5-0 Prolene in a 2-layer running fashion. We checked pulses at the end of the procedure. We had nice Doppler on the radial and ulnar, the palmar arch, and each digital arteries of the left hand; there was good capillary refill. The wound was irrigated, and subcutaneous tissues were closed with interrupted sutures of 3-0 Vicryl after ensuring that hemostasis was present. This skin was closed with 4-0 Vicryl running in subcuticular fashion. Dermabond was applied as the dressing. The patient went to the recovery room in stable condition.

98. OPERATIVE REPORT

PREOPERATIVE DIAGNOSIS: Umbilical hernia.

POSTOPERATIVE DIAGNOSIS: Umbilical hernia.

PROCEDURE PERFORMED: Umbilical hernia repair, 10.2 cm with mesh.

ANESTHESIA: General anesthesia.

OPERATIVE NOTE: With the patient under general anesthesia, the abdomen was prepped and draped in a sterile manner. A standard skin line incision just below the umbilicus was made with sharp dissection carried down to the fascia. The umbilicus was freed from the underlying hernia, which contained some fatty material. We did not enter the peritoneal sac at any time. We were able to free up the fascial edge all the way around using sharp dissection and electrocautery. We were then able to reduce the herniated fat through the fascial opening, and then we closed the fascial opening using interrupted 0 Vicryl. Once this was closed, we did take a patch of Prolene mesh and placed it on top of our repair and tacked that around circumferentially with some additional 0 Vicryl. With this accomplished, hemostasis was in place. We then tacked the umbilicus back to the fascia using a 2-0 Vicryl and then closed the subcutaneous tissue using 3-0 chromic and skin using 4-0 Vicryl in a subcuticular manner. Steri-Strips were applied, and we did place part of a cotton ball into the umbilicus for shape, and then a sterile dressing was applied. The patient tolerated the procedure well and was discharged from the recovery area in stable condition. At the end of the procedure, all sponges and instruments were accounted for.

99. OPERATIVE REPORT

PREOPERATIVE DIAGNOSIS: Recurrent carcinoma of the prostate.

POSTOPERATIVE DIAGNOSIS: Recurrent carcinoma of the prostate.

PROCEDURE PERFORMED: Cryoablation of the prostate.

CLINICAL NOTE: This is a 53-year-old gentleman who has undergone radiation therapy for adenocarcinoma of the prostate. Unfortunately, he developed problems again and underwent a needle biopsy, and recurrence of his cancer was found. Options were discussed with the patient, and he has opted to proceed with cryoablation. He has been told of the risk of incontinence and possible rectal injury. He understands and still chooses to proceed with the surgery.

PROCEDURE: The patient was given a general endotracheal anesthetic and was prepped and draped in the lithotomy position. An 18-French Foley catheter was placed in the bladder. A transrectal probe was introduced. Prostate volume was returned at 27.5 g. A six-probe freeze was selected. Using quick stick method, sheaths were placed using ultrasound guidance. Following placement of the sheaths, temperature probes were then placed in the left and right neurovascular bundles, apex, external sphincter, and Denonvilliers fascia. A two-cycle probe freeze was performed. The first cycle was a very rapid freeze, and the second cycle was a more prolonged freeze. The external sphincter temperature never reached less than 0° C. The freeze was monitored both digitally and radiographically with ultrasound. The probes were then withdrawn after the full thaw. Two active thaw cycles were undertaken. The perineal incisions were then closed with 3-0 plain catgut subcuticular sutures. The catheter was left in. The patient tolerated the procedure well and was transferred to the recovery room in good condition.

100. PSYCHOLOGICAL EVALUATION

HISTORY: Mr. Meyer is a 48-year-old, divorced, white male who was admitted after he was found lying on the floor in his apartment. Evidently, he had taken a fall, and he had some bruises on his face and tongue. Later, during the hospitalization, he developed delirium tremens and was required to go on the ventilator. Earlier this week, I also came to see this patient, but at that time, he was given a dose of Haldol, and he was quite drowsy and sleepy.

Today, I reviewed his medical records and also met with the patient for a full evaluation. He was fairly cooperative. According to the nursing staff, the patient was just transferred to the rehab hospital, but there he became non-responsive and was transferred back yesterday. During this meeting, actually, he was pretty awake, although his concentration was still somewhat poor, but he seemed a fairly good historian. As I approached the patient, he was immediately able to recognize me, saying that I saw him many years back for "mental capacity" for Social Security benefits. At that time also, the patient had a history of auditory and visual hallucinations. The patient still talks about the same symptoms, saying he is seeing different animals from the side of his eyes and that it becomes quite scary; he will see elephants, people being hanged, and when he sees these things, he gets very nervous. He also talks about having auditory hallucinations.

Again, the patient corroborated that it is nothing new and it has been going on for a number of years. He has been treated with Trazodone and then with some other medication like Mellaril, but all it did was make his mouth dry. Surprisingly, related to these psychotic symptoms, he never has had any psychiatric hospitalizations.

Today, the patient also admitted that he is feeling quite depressed, and he does not feel good. He has hopelessness and worthlessness feelings, but did add that he will not hurt or kill himself. Because of pain, he complains of sleep difficulties. He does get angry and irritable because the staff tries to be smart with him; like yesterday, he was talking about not eating and still they would keep on bringing food to him. However, the patient denies if he is physically aggressive to anyone. Then I also confronted the patient about his drinking habits, but the patient said it is just a rumor, saying he is not using any alcohol or street drugs, and he has no idea who is putting it in his records. He does complain of significant anxiety symptoms also.

PAST MEDICAL HISTORY: Significant for hypertension, gout, hypercalcemia, and now general debility. His previous coronary angiogram was negative.

MEDICATIONS: At the time of admission, the patient was on numerous medications, but now they had been cut down significantly.

PAST PSYCHIATRIC HISTORY: As above. He does have a history of psychosis, but questionable treatment.

FAMILY HISTORY: The patient tells me he comes from a very large family. There were 11 kids. Some of his brothers are deceased. He could not really tell me if any other brother or sister has a diagnosis of psychosis. Both of his parents are deceased. The patient has two children; both of them are doing very well—one is a teacher and another a technician in a hospital.

PERSONAL AND SOCIAL HISTORY: The patient was married. His marriage lasted for about 9 years. For many years, he worked on trenches. The patient minimizes if he abuses alcohol and denies using any street drugs.

MENTAL STATUS EXAMINATION: This is a heavyset male. He was pretty cooperative. He was able to recognize the undersigned right away. He remembered the name. His mood is quite depressed. He is close to tears often. Affect is flat. He also seems quite nervous. His voice is somewhat shaky. The patient was able to give his birthday month and the year correctly and knew he was 48 years old. The patient knew he was in the hospital and who the president of the United States is. He was off on current time with the serial 7's. He was not able to spell the word "money" and had quite a hard time spelling it backwards. He continues to have both auditory and visual hallucinations and some paranoid behavior. No acute agitation or aggression.

ASSESSMENT:

1. Psychotic disorder, NOS. It does seem functional, especially with such a long history, and possibly, there is worsening of the symptoms with underlying delirium earlier.

RECOMMENDATIONS: Today, I tried to go into my old files, but I was unable to find the evaluation that I completed for the Social Security office. Looking at his current picture, the patient does seem quite psychotic, and I think it is reasonable to treat him with any antipsychotics. Probably, he could benefit from a trial with antidepressants also, but I would hold using too many medications suddenly at this point, especially, as his physical status is so unclear. It does not seem there is any explanation why he was so unresponsive just yesterday. Targeting his psychosis, we will start him on Risperdal small dose and slowly go up on the dose tolerated.

Thank you for asking me to see this interesting patient in consultation.

APPENDIX B

Answers to Odd-Numbered Workbook Questions

NOTE: The following reference manuals were used in preparing these answers: *2025 ICD-10-CM, 2025 ICD-10-PCS, 2024 HCPCS Level II,* and *Current Procedural Terminology, 2025.*

CHAPTER 1: REIMBURSEMENT, HIPAA, AND COMPLIANCE

Theory

1. a. persons eligible for disability benefits from Social Security
   b. persons with permanent kidney failure requiring dialysis or transplant
3. Social Security Administration
5. 80%
7. 12
9. OBRA
11. beneficiaries
13. Medicare Advantage
15. Administrative Simplification
17. National Provider
19. limiting
21. Internet Only
23. Staff
25. Program, All-Inclusive

CHAPTER 2: AN OVERVIEW OF ICD-10-CM

Theory

1. True
3. True
5. False
7. False

9. True
11. False
13. True
15. b
17. e
19. c

Practical

21. aneurysm (cirsoid) (false) (ruptured)
23. Diseases of the Circulatory System
25. Rheumatic fever with heart involvement
27. acute pericarditis not specified as rheumatic (I30.-)
29. abscess
31. pain
33. mass
35. dwarfism
37. fatigue
39. positive

CHAPTER 3: ICD-10-CM OUTPATIENT CODING AND REPORTING GUIDELINES

Theory

1. False
3. False
5. True
7. False
9. False
11. True
13. True
15. False

Practical

17. Congestive heart failure, **I50.9**. The shortness of breath is a symptom of congestive heart failure and is not reported.
19. Hypertension with end stage renal disease, **I12.0**; end stage renal disease, **N18.6**. There is a combination code for hypertension with end stage renal disease. **I12.0** assumes a causal relationship in this scenario. Under code **I12.0** in the Tabular, a notation states "Use additional code to identify the stage of chronic kidney disease (**N18.5**, **N18.6**)."
21. COPD with acute lower respiratory infection, **J44.0**
23. Exposure to tuberculosis, **Z20.1**
25. Abnormal perfusion study, **R94.39**; cardiovascular disease, **I25.1**0. The purpose of the visit is the abnormal perfusion study; therefore it is reported first, followed by the cardiovascular disease.
27. Contusion of the left cheek, **S00.83XA**; fist fight, **Y04.0XXA**. External cause codes are never reported as a first-listed diagnosis.

29. Encounter for insulin pump titration, **Z46.81**
31. Infant, liveborn, twin, born in hospital, **Z38.30**
33. Abrasion of left upper arm, **S40.812A**
35. Acute bronchitis, **J20.9**; COPD, **J44.0**; cigarette smoker, **F17.210**. If the infectious organism is known, it would also be reported.

CHAPTER 4: USING ICD-10-CM

Theory

1. False
3. False
5. True
7. True
9. False
11. False
13. False
15. False
17. Heartburn, acid regurgitation, belching, hoarseness in the morning, reflux, pain in chest, trouble swallowing, choking feeling, dry cough
19. Swelling, pain, discoloration, disfiguration
21. Residual: Constrictive pericarditis
    Cause: Tuberculosis infection

Practical

23. **J01.90** (Sinusitis, acute), **J32.9** (Sinusitis [chronic])
25. **J62.8** (Pneumoconiosis, dust, lime)
27. **J14** (Pneumonia, in, *Hemophilus influenzae*)
29. **I95.9** (Hypotension)
31. **K85.90** (Pancreatitis), **K86.1** (Pancreatitis, chronic)
33. **E83.31, M90.80** (Rickets, vitamin-D-resistant)
35. **K70.11** (Ascites, due to, hepatitis, alcoholic), **F10.288** (Dependence, alcohol, with, specified disorder NEC)

CHAPTER 5: CHAPTER-SPECIFIC GUIDELINES (ICD-10-CM CHAPTERS 1-10)

Theory

1. True
3. True
5. False
7. True
9. True
11. True
13. True
15. True
17. False
19. True

Practical

21. **A41.9** (Sepsis [generalized]), **R65.20** (Sepsis, severe), **N17.9** (Failure, renal, acute), **J96.00** (Failure, respiration, respiratory, acute)
23. **E86.0** (Dehydration), **B19.10** (Hepatitis, B)
25. **J85.2** (Abscess, lung), **B95.62** (Infection, bacterial, as cause of disease classified elsewhere, *Staphylococcus, aureus*, methicillin resistant [MRSA])
27. **Z09** (Examination, follow-up [routine] [following], surgery NEC), **Q54.9** (Hypospadias). Because this follow-up exam is part of the episode of care in which surgery corrected the hypospadias, the hypospadias is still coded as if it is an active disease. Once all treatment for the surgery is complete, a history of hypospadias would be reported instead.
29. **C80.0** (Table of Neoplasms: Neoplasm, disseminated, Primary), **R18.0** (Ascites, malignant)
31. **L03.116** (Cellulitis, lower limb), **E11.65** (Diabetes, type 2, with, hyperglycemia)
33. **O9A.111** (Pregnancy, complicated by, neoplasm, malignant), **C50.912** (Table of Neoplasms: Neoplasm, breast, Primary)
35. **C61** (Table of Neoplasms: Neoplasm, prostate, Primary), **D63.0** (Anemia, in, neoplastic disease)
37. **K56.609** (Obstruction, intestine), **I12.0** (Hypertension, kidney, with stage 5 chronic kidney disease), **N18.5** (Disease, kidney, chronic, hypertensive, stage 5)
39. **C79.31** (Table of Neoplasms: Neoplasm, brain NEC, Secondary), **Z85.3** (History, personal [of], malignant neoplasm, breast), **Z90.12** (Absence, breast(s) [acquired])
41. **D45** (Polycythemia, vera)
43. **T85.614A** (Complication[s], insulin pump, mechanical, breakdown), **T38.3X1A** (Table of Drugs and Chemicals, Insulin, Poisoning, Accidental [unintentional]), **E10.641** (Diabetes, with, hypoglycemia, with coma), **E16.A3** (Hypoglycemia, level, 3)
45. **C34.11** (Table of Neoplasms: Neoplasm, lung, upper lobe, Primary)
47. **I21.3** (Infarct, myocardium [acute], Q wave)
49. **F20.9** (Schizophrenia, Schizophrenic), **F91.9** (Disorder, conduct [childhood]), **Z91.148** (Noncompliance, with, medication regimen)
51. **B05.1** (Meningitis, in [due to], measles)
53. **A52.15** (Polyneuropathy, in [due to], syphilis [late]), **A52.77** (Syphilis, joint [late])
55. **G80.2** (Palsy, cerebral, hemiplegic, spastic)
57. **H81.09** (Meniere's disease, syndrome or vertigo)
59. **I50.1** (Failure, ventricle, left), **Z99.11** (Dependence, on, ventilator)

Reports

61. Report 9: **C50.111** (Table of Neoplasms: Neoplasm, breast, central portion, Primary)
63. Report 20: **C79.82** (Table of Neoplasms: Neoplasm, endocervix, Secondary), **C80.1** (Table of Neoplasms: Neoplasm, unknown site or unspecified, Primary)
65. Report 39: **E66.01** (Obesity, morbid), **K76.0** (Fatty, liver NEC), **Z68.42** (Body, mass index, adult, 45.0–49.9)

67. Report 42: **H02.411** (Blepharoptosis, mechanical), **H53.461** (Hemianopia, homonymous)
69. Report 90: **C61** (Table of Neoplasms: Neoplasm, prostate [gland], Primary)

CHAPTER 6: CHAPTER-SPECIFIC GUIDELINES (ICD-10-CM CHAPTERS 11-14)

Theory

1. True
3. True
5. False
7. False
9. True

Practical

11. **K03.2** (Erosion, dental [idiopathic] [occupational] [due to diet, drugs, or vomiting])
13. **N83.6** (Hemorrhage, fallopian tube)
15. **N76.4** (Cellulitis, genital organ, female [external])
17. **N47.2** (Paraphimosis [congenital])
19. **N91.1** (Amenorrhea, secondary)
21. **M79.81** (Hematoma, nontraumatic, soft tissue)
23. **K51.412** (Polyp, polypus, colon, inflammatory, with, intestinal obstruction)
25. **L97.112** (Ulcer, lower limb, thigh, right, with, exposed fat layer)
27. **K40.41** (Hernia, inguinal [internal], with, gangrene, recurrent)
29. **N03.1** (Nephritis, nephritic [focal], chronic, with, focal and segmental glomerular lesions)
31. **L05.02** (Sinus, pilonidal, with abscess)
33. **M60.162** (Myositis, interstitial, lower leg)
35. **M32.13** (Lupus, erythematosus, systemic, with organ or system involvement, lung)
37. **M00.242** (Arthritis, streptococcal, hand joint), **B95.1** (*Streptococcus*, group, B, as cause of disease classified elsewhere)
39. **M60.221** (Granuloma, foreign body, upper arm)
41. **N61.1** (Abscess, areola [chronic])

Reports

43. Report 6: **L90.5** (Scar)
45. Report 10: **S14.151A** (Injury, spinal [cord], cervical [neck], posterior cord syndrome, C1 level), **S12.000A** (Fracture, traumatic, neck, cervical vertebra, first [displaced]), **S12.100A** (Fracture, traumatic, neck, cervical vertebra, second [displaced]), **S12.200A** (Fracture, traumatic, neck, cervical vertebra, third [displaced]), **S12.300A** (Fracture, traumatic, neck, cervical vertebra, fourth [displaced]),**V47.0XXA** (External Cause Index, Accident, transport, car occupant, driver, collision [with], stationary object, non-traffic)
47. Report 12: **L89.224** (Ulcer, pressure, hip)

49. Report 14: **M60.812** (Myositis), **Z99.11** (Dependence, on ventilator)
51. Report 31: **K63.5** (Polyp, colon)
53. Report 33: **N49.3** (Disease, Fournier [gangrene]), **T18.2XXA** (Foreign body, entering through orifice, stomach)
55. Report 38: **R32** (Incontinence), **Z85.46** (History, personal, malignant neoplasm, prostate)
57. Report 43: **M51.16** (Displacement, intervertebral disc, lumbar region, with neuritis, radiculitis, radiculopathy, or sciatica)
59. Report 92: **N20.0** (Calculus, kidney)

CHAPTER 7: CHAPTER-SPECIFIC GUIDELINES (ICD-10-CM CHAPTERS 15-21)

Theory

1. True
3. True
5. True
7. True
9. False
11. False
13. True
15. True
17. anomaly
19. abnormal
21. third degree
23. 18
25. severity

Practical

27. **S40.812A** (Abrasion, arm [upper])
29. **T78.2XXA** (Shock, anaphylactic)
31. **O00.90** (Pregnancy, ectopic [ruptured]), **O08.0** (Peritonitis, following ectopic or molar pregnancy)
33. **Q55.64** (Concealed penis)
35. **O26.53** (Pregnancy, complicated by, hypotension), **Z3A.32** (Pregnancy, weeks of gestation, 32 weeks)
37. **R13.0** (Aphagia)
39. **S93.402A** (Sprain, ankle)
41. **T23.201D** (Burn, hand[s], right, second degree)
43. **R80.1** (Proteinuria, persistent)
45. **S00.33XD** (Contusion, nose)
47. **Q99.2** (Syndrome, fragile X)
49. **O30.203** (Pregnancy, complicated by, multiple gestations, quadruplet) **Z3A.30** (Pregnancy, weeks of gestation, 30 weeks)
51. **T43.1X1A** (Table of Drugs and Chemicals, Monoamine oxidase inhibitor NEC, Poisoning, Accidental [unintentional], **G25.1** (Tremor[s], drug induced)
53. **S60.821A** (Blister, wrist)

55. **S42.001G** (Fracture, traumatic clavicle)
57. **R06.03** (Distress, respiratory), **R53.83** (Fatigue)

Reports

59. Report 28: **O76** (Delivery, complicated, by, fetal, heart rate or rhythm), **O66.0** (Delivery, complicated, by, obstructed labor, due to, dystocia, due to, shoulder), **O70.1** (Delivery, complicated, by, laceration, perineum, second degree), **Z3A.38** (Pregnancy, weeks of gestation, 38 weeks), **Z37.0** (Outcome of delivery, single liveborn)
61. Report 40: **T15.01XA** (Foreign body, cornea)
63. Report 95: **M25.551** (Pain[s], joint, hip), **R05.8** (Cough, specified)

CHAPTER 8: INTRODUCTION TO CPT

Theory

1-4. any of the following: service or procedure, anatomic site, condition or disease, synonym, eponym, abbreviation
5. d
7. b
9. Radiology
11. American Medical Association, or AMA
13. stand-alone code
15. CPT codes and/or HCPCS codes
17. 1966
19. Health Insurance Portability and Accountability Act, or HIPAA

Practical

Radiology

21. **77799**
23. **77499**

Pathology and Laboratory

25. **81099**

Medicine

27. **96999**

CHAPTER 9: INTRODUCTION TO THE LEVEL II NATIONAL CODES (HCPCS)

Theory

1-4. any of the following: procedures, supplies, products, services
5. Alpha-Numeric
7. Professional
9. G
11. Q
13. EY
15. Q
17. d

19. e
21. b

Practical

23. **J0129**
25. **A4680**
27. **V5264**
29. **E0969**
31. **G0009**

CHAPTER 10: MODIFIERS

Theory

1. A
3. preoperative services/management or preop
5. no

Practical

7. -50, **M71.21** (Cyst, Baker's), **M71.22** (Cyst, Baker's)
9. -53, **M17.9** (Osteoarthritis, knee), **I95.89** (Hypotension), **Z53.09** (Procedure, not done, because of, contraindication)
11. -32, **K50.10** (Enteritis, regional, large intestine [colon] [rectum])
13. -32, **Z02.6** (Examination, medical, insurance purposes)
15. -76
17. -99
19. -55
21. -FA

CHAPTER 11: EVALUATION AND MANAGEMENT (E/M) SERVICES

Theory

1. c
3. a
5. e
7. b
9. high
11. low
13. elements
15. moderate severity
17. self-limited/minor severity
19. face-to-face or direct, non face-to-face
21. counseling
23. emergency
25. critical care
27. transfer of care

Practical

Office or Other Outpatient Services and Hospital Inpatient Services

29. a. minimal, minimal/none
    b. minimal
    c. straightforward
    d. **99202**
31. **99222** (Evaluation and Management, Hospital)
33. **99223** (Hospital Services, Inpatient Services, Initial Hospital Care), **I21.19** (Infarction, myocardium, ST elevation inferior), **I25.10** (Arteriosclerosis, coronary [artery]), **Z95.5** (Status, angioplasty, coronary artery, with implant)
35. **99231** (Hospital Services, Inpatient Services, Subsequent Hospital Care), **J15.9** (Pneumonia, bacterial)

Consultation Services

37. **99244** (Consultation, Office and/or Other Outpatient), **R10.2** (Pain, pelvic [female]), **N94.10** (Dyspareunia [female])

    Note: All three key components must be met for the service to qualify for the higher level code. In this case, only the MDM complexity was of a higher level, requiring the choice of the lower-level code.
39. **99253** (New Patient, Inpatient Consultations)
41. **99232** (Hospital Inpatient Services, Subsequent Hospital Care), **R21** (Rash)

    Note that adverse effect from a drug would not be reported as the physician is looking for another cause.
43. **99231** (Hospital Inpatient Services, Subsequent Hospital Care), **G44.209** (Headache, tension)
45. **99242** (Consultation, Office and/or Other Outpatient, New or Established Patient), **K41.91** (Hernia, femoral, recurrent)
47. **99245** (Consultation, Office and/or Other Outpatient, New or Established Patient), **M51.06** (Disorder, disc, with myelopathy, lumbar region)

Emergency Department Services, Nursing Facility, and Home Services

49. **99283** (Established Patient, Emergency Department Services), **S52.539A** (Colles', fracture), **W21.89XA** (External Cause Index, Striking against, other sports equipment), **Y93.64** (External Cause Index, Activity, baseball)
51. **99342** (Home Services, New Patient), **R60.0** (Edema, legs)

    Note that the leg pain is not reported because the medical documentation indicated that the pain was due to the edema.
53. **99309** (Nursing Facility Services, Subsequent Care), **R41.0** (Confusion), **R42** (Dizziness), **I69.30** (Sequelae, infarction, cerebral)
55. **99304** (Nursing Facility Services, Initial Care)

Prolonged Services and Preventive Medicine Services

57. **99205** for the office visit (Office and/or Other Outpatient Services, New Patient) and **99417 x 2** for Prolonged Services (Prolonged Services)

Services From Throughout the E/M Section

59. **99205** (Office and/or Other Outpatient Services, Office Visit, New Patient)
61. **99234** (Discharge Services, Observation Care), **L29.89** (Pruritus, specified NEC), **R06.02** (Short, breath), **T39.95XA** (Table of Drugs and Chemicals, Analgesic, Adverse Effect)
63. **99252** (Consultation, Inpatient)
65. **99291** (Critical Care Services, Evaluation and Management), **99292 x 3** (Critical Care Services, Evaluation and Management), **J96.90** (Failure, respiratory), **I50.9** (Failure, heart), **J44.1** (Disease, pulmonary chronic obstructive, with exacerbation [acute]), **Z99.11** (Dependence, on, ventilator)

Reports

67. Report 1: **99284** (Evaluation and Management, Emergency Department), **O23.43** (Infection, urinary, complicating, pregnancy), **N39.0** (Infection, urinary [tract]), **R60.0** (Edema, legs), **Z3A.36** (Pregnancy, weeks of gestation, 36 weeks)
69. Report 3: **99212** (Evaluation and Management, Office and Other Outpatient), **S93.401A** (Sprain, ankle)
71. Report 5: **99231** (Evaluation and Management, Hospital)

CHAPTER 12: ANESTHESIA

Theory

1. moderate sedation or conscious sedation
3. base unit
5. preoperative services
7. conversion

Practical

9. P4 (A patient with severe systemic disease that is a constant threat to life)
11. P3 (A patient with severe systemic disease)
13. P2 (A patient with mild systemic disease)
15. **01382** (Anesthesia, Knee)
17. **00144** (Anesthesia, Corneal Transplant)
19. **00124** (Anesthesia, Otoscopy)
21. **01920-P2** (Anesthesia, Cardiac Catheterization)
23. **K57.33** (Diverticulitis, intestine, large, with, bleeding)
25. **E05.01** (Hyperthyroidism, with, goiter, with thyroid storm)

Reports

27. Report 7: **00400** (Anesthesia, Arm, Upper)
29. Report 44: **00140** (Anesthesia, Eye), **99100** (Anesthesia Special Circumstances, Extreme Age)

CHAPTER 13: SURGERY GUIDELINES AND GENERAL SURGERY

Theory

1. Female Genital
3. categories
5. unlisted
7. major
9. yes
11. local
13. general
15. **99070**
17. same
19. dehiscence

Practical

21. **10004-69990**
23. Operating
25. **42400**
27. therapeutic
29. **40799**

CHAPTER 14: INTEGUMENTARY SYSTEM

Theory

Integumentary System Terminology

1. b
3. i
5. a
7. f
9. c
11. a
13. i
15. c
17. e
19. f
21. d

Practical

23. **12032** (Repair, Wound, Intermediate), **99070** (Special Services, Supply of Materials), **S41.101A** (Wound, open, arm, [upper])

    Note: You do not report an E/M code because this is an established patient and the treatment constitutes the main service provided to the patient.

25. **19081-LT** (Breast, Biopsy, with Localization Device Placement, Stereotactic Guidance), **99070** (Special Services, Supply of Materials), **D48.62** (Table of Neoplasms: Neoplasm, breast, Uncertain Behavior)

    Note: You do not report an E/M code because this is an established patient and the treatment constitutes the main service provided to the patient.
27. **11451** (Hidradenitis, Excision), **L73.2** (Hidradenitis)
29. **11971** (Removal, Tissue Expander)
31. **11976** (Removal, Implant, Contraceptive Capsules), **Z30.46** (Contraception, maintenance, subdermal implantable)
33. **11444** (Excision, Skin, Lesion, Benign) for 4 cm face lesion, **11423-51** (Excision, Skin, Lesion, Benign) for 3 cm neck lesion, **D23.30** (Table of Neoplasms: Neoplasm, skin, face NOS, Benign), **D23.4** (Table of Neoplasms: Neoplasm, skin, neck, Benign)
35. **17000** (Destruction, Lesion, Facial), **17003** x **2** (Destruction, Lesion, Facial), **L57.0** (Keratosis, actinic)
37. **12035** (Wound, Repair, Legs, Intermediate); **11042-51** (Debridement, Subcutaneous Tissue), **S81.801A** (Wound, open, leg [lower]), **W09.1XXA** (External Cause Index, Fall, from, off, playground equipment, swing), **W27.1XXA** (External Cause Index Contact with, garden, fork), **Y92.830** (External Cause Index, Place of occurrence, park [public])
39. **17110** (Destruction, Warts, Flat), **B07.8** (Wart, Flat)
41. **11000, 11001** (Debridement, Skin, Eczematous), **L30.9** (Eczema)
43. **16000** (Burns, Initial Treatment), **T23.169A** (Burn, dorsum of hand, first degree), **T31.0** (Burn, extent, less than 10 percent), **X16.XXXA** (External Cause Index, Burning, steam, pipe), **Y92.009** (External Cause Index, Place of occurrence, residence)
45. **19020** (Mastotomy, Drainage of Abscess), **N61.1** (Abscess, breast)

Reports

47. Report 7: **21931** (Excision, Tumor, Back/Flank, 3 cm or greater), **D17.1** (Lipoma, site classification, trunk, [skin])

    Note: **11406** would not be correct because the report indicates "dissected free of the muscle."
49. Report 9: **19120-RT** (Excision, Breast, Lesion), **C50.111** (Table of Neoplasms: Neoplasm, breast, central portion, Primary)
51. Report 12: **15940** (Ulcer, Pressure), **L89.224** (Ulcer, pressure, hip)

    Note: Modifier -22 may be added to **15940** due to the extensive size of the ulcer.

CHAPTER 15: MUSCULOSKELETAL SYSTEM

Theory

Musculoskeletal Terminology

1. d
3. j
5. b
7. c
9. h
11. g

Answer the Following

13. aspiration of a joint
15. fascia lata graft
17. arthroscopy
19. No, the removal is part of the cast service.
21. The primary difference is extent. The codes in the musculoskeletal system subsection are of biopsies of deep subcutaneous tissue, muscle, and/or bone, whereas the codes in the integumentary system subsection are for skin and subcutaneous tissue.

Practical

23. **29075-58** (Cast, Elbow to Finger), **Z46.89** (Admission [for], orthopedic [cast]), **S52.119D** (Fracture, traumatic, radius, upper end, torus)
25. **28406** (Fracture, Calcaneus, with Manipulation), **S92.009A** (Fracture, traumatic, tarsal, bone[s], calcaneus)
27. **26700** (Metacarpophalangeal Joint, Dislocation, Closed Treatment), **S63.269A** (Dislocation, finger, metacarpophalangeal)
29. **27520** (Fracture, Patella, Closed Treatment, without Manipulation), **S82.009A** (Fracture, traumatic, patella)
31. **27570** (Manipulation, Knee), **S83.116A** (Dislocation, knee, proximal tibia, anteriorly)
33. **21343** (Sinuses, Frontal, Fracture, Open Treatment)
35. **20615** (Aspiration, Cyst, Bone)
37. **20822** (Replantation, Digit)
39. **20526** (Injection, Carpal Tunnel, Therapeutic), **G56.00** (Syndrome, carpal tunnel)
41. **20665** (Removal, Halo)
43. **21450** (Fracture, Mandible, Closed Treatment, without Manipulation)
45. **29750** (Cast, Wedging)
47. **29520** (Strapping, Hip)
49. **29200** (Strapping, Thorax)
51. **29049** (Cast, Ambulatory, Figure-of-eight Shoulder)
53. **29860** (Arthroscopy, Diagnostic, Hip)
55. **29877** (Arthroscopy, Surgical, Knee)
57. **29848** (Ligament, Release, Transverse Carpal)
59. **21032** (Excision, Maxillary, Torus Palatinus)

Reports

61. Report 13: **20610-LT** (Injection, Joint), **M75.102** (Syndrome, rotator cuff, shoulder)
63. Report 15: **25606-LT** (Fracture, Radius, Distal), **S52.572A** (Fracture, traumatic, radius, lower end, intraarticular NEC), **W10.9XXA** (External Cause Index, Fall, from, unspecified, stairs and steps, initial encounter)
65. Report 17: **27244** or **27244-RT** (Fracture, Femur, Subtrochanteric, Plate/Screw Implant), **S72.21XA** (Fracture, traumatic, femur, upper end, subtrochanteric [displaced])

CHAPTER 16: RESPIRATORY SYSTEM

Theory

Respiratory Terminology

1. d
3. k
5. b
7. c
9. f
11. m
13. a
15. e

Answer the Following

17. nasal button
19. septoplasty
21. posterior
23. transtracheal and cricothyroid
25. 50

Practical

27. **31267** (Antrostomy, Sinus, Maxillary)
29. **31628-RT** (Bronchoscopy, Biopsy), **31632-RT** (Bronchoscopy, Biopsy). Note: Code **31628** is for a single lobe and two lobes were biopsied. Code **31632** is an add-on code reporting the biopsy of the additional lobe.
31. **31575** (Laryngoscopy, Flexible, Diagnostic)
33. **30801** (Ablation, Turbinate Mucosa). Note: Code specified unilateral or bilateral.
35. **30115** and **30115-50** (Excision, Nose, Polyp)
37. **31536** (Laryngoscopy, Direct)
39. **31400** (Arytenoidectomy)
41. **31720** (Aspiration, Trachea, Nasotracheal)
43. **31830** (Revision, Tracheostomy, Scar)
45. **32658** (Thoracoscopy, Surgical)
47. **32800** (Hernia Repair, Lung)
49. **30930** (Fracture, Nasal Turbinate, Therapeutic)
51. **31613** (Tracheostoma, Revision), **J95.02** (Tracheostomy, complication, infection), **L03.221** (Cellulitis, neck [region])
53. **32440** (Pneumonectomy), **J61** (Asbestosis [occupational])
55. **32900** (Ribs, Resection), **Q76.6** (Deformity, rib, congenital)
57. **32560** (Pleurodesis, Instillation of Agent), **C56.9** (Table of Neoplasms: Neoplasm, ovary, Primary), **J91.0** (Effusion, pleura, malignant)

Reports

59. Report 19: **32480-LT** (Lobectomy, Lung), **32225-LT** (Decortication, Lung, with Partial), **J85.2** (Abscess, lung)
61. Report 23: **32555** (Thoracentesis, with Imaging Guidance), **J90** (Effusion, pleura)

CHAPTER 17: CARDIOVASCULAR SYSTEM

Theory

Cardiovascular Terminology

1. e
3. b
5. d
7. a
9. i
11. f
13. j
15. d
17. i
19. h
21. n
23. b
25. l

Answer the Following

27. internally or externally, or intracardiac or external
29. epicardial and transvenous
31. No, suture removal is bundled into the pacemaker procedure.
33. 24
35. patient-activated event recorder
37. reversible
39. embolus

Practical

41. **33390** (Valvuloplasty, Aortic Valve)
43. **33464** (Tricuspid Valve, Repair)
45. **93000** (Electrocardiography, Evaluation)
47. **92920** (Angioplasty, Coronary Artery, Percutaneous Transluminal)
49. **93010** (Electrocardiography, Evaluation)
51. **37609** (Ligation, Artery, Temporal)
53. **37246** (Angioplasty, Aorta, Intraoperative)
55. **33513** (Bypass Graft, Venous, Coronary), **I24.89** (Insufficiency, coronary [acute or subacute])
57. **33967** (Balloon Assisted Device, Aorta), **I21.9** (Infarction, myocardium, myocardial [acute]), **R57.0** (Shock, cardiogenic)
59. **33641** (Repair, Heart, Septal Defect, Atrium), **Q21.10** (Defect, septal, atrial)
61. **33533** (Bypass Graft, Arterial, Coronary), **33517** (Coronary Artery Bypass Graft, Arterial-Venous), **33530** (Reoperation, Coronary Artery Bypass, Valve Procedure), **I25.10** (Arteriosclerosis, coronary [artery])

Reports

63. Report 26: **33533** (Coronary Artery Bypass Graft, Arterial Bypass), **I25.10** (Arteriosclerosis, coronary [artery]), **I51.9** (Dysfunction, ventricular)

65. Report 96: **93312-26** (Transesophageal, Doppler Echocardiography), **I35.0** (Stenosis, aortic [valve])

CHAPTER 18: HEMIC, LYMPHATIC, MEDIASTINUM, AND DIAPHRAGM

Theory

Hemic and Lymphatic Terminology

1. k
3. e
5. g
7. d
9. i
11. c
13. f
15. b
17. h
19. c

Mediastinum and Diaphragm Terminology

21. m
23. j
25. d
27. l
29. k
31. g
33. b

Practical

35. **38720-LT** (Lymphadenectomy, Radical, Cervical), **C77.0** (Table of Neoplasms: Neoplasm, lymph, gland, cervical, Secondary), **C50.012** (Table of Neoplasms: Neoplasm, breast, nipple, Primary)

    Note: The lymph gland neoplasm is first-listed because it was the reason for the procedure.
37. **38241** (Bone Marrow, T-Cell Transplantation), **C92.00** (Leukemia, myelogenous)
39. **38230** (Harvesting, Bone Marrow, Allogeneic), **Z52.3** (Donor, bone, marrow)
41. **39200** (Resection, Cyst, Mediastinal)
43. **38209** (Transplantation, Stem Cells, Washing)
45. **78195-26** (Nuclear Medicine, Lymph Nodes), **38792-59** (Lymphadenectomy, Injection, Sentinel Node), **38530** (Excision, Lymph Nodes)

CHAPTER 19: DIGESTIVE SYSTEM

Theory

Digestive Terminology

1. b
3. f

5. g
7. a
9. i
11. i
13. e
15. h
17. a

Practical

19. **43194** (Endoscopy, Esophagus, Removal, Foreign Body)
21. **43410** (Suture, Esophagus, Wound)
23. **44345** (Colostomy, Revision)
25. **42104** (Excision, Lesion, Palate)
27. **42831** (Adenoids, Excision)
29. **49521** (Repair, Hernia, Inguinal)
31. **40650** (Repair, Lip)
33. **42507** (Parotid Duct, Diversion)
35. **43605** (Biopsy, Stomach)
37. **44604** (Suture, Intestines, Large, Wound)
39. **49320** (Laparoscopy, Diagnostic)
41. **99285-25** (Evaluation and Management, Emergency Department), **43752** (Tube Placement, Nasogastric Tube), **K92.0** (Hematemesis), **R18.8** (Ascites [abdominal]), **D62** (Anemia, due to, blood loss, acute)

Reports

43. Report 31: **45384** (Colonoscopy, Removal, Flexible, Polyp), **K63.5** (Polyp, colon)

    Note: The entry listed under "Neoplasm, intestine, cecum, Benign" indicates **K63.5**, the same code as for the benign polyp of the colon, and the code is only reported once.
45. Report 33: **44143** (Hartmann Procedure, Open), **43500-51** (Gastrotomy, Foreign Body Removal), **43830** (Gastrostomy, temporary), **N49.3** (Disease, Fournier [gangrene]); **T18.2XXA** (Foreign body, entering through orifice, stomach)
47. Report 35: **43752** (Orogastric Tube Placement), **K31.84** (Gastroparesis)
49. Report 98: **49617** (Repair, Hernia, Umbilical, Reducible), **K42.9** (Hernia, umbilical)

CHAPTER 20: URINARY AND MALE GENITAL SYSTEMS

Theory

Urinary System Terminology

1. d
3. g
5. f
7. k
9. c
11. l

13. i
15. a
17. d
19. f
21. b
23. h

Male Genital Terminology

25. c
27. e
29. b
31. d
33. e
35. f
37. i
39. c
41. c
43. a
45. f
47. a
49. d
51. e
53. a
55. d
57. c

Practical

59. **50390** (Aspiration, Cyst, Kidney), **N28.1** (Cyst, kidney, solitary, acquired)
61. **52450** (Incision, Prostate, Transurethral), **N41.1** (Prostatitis, hypertrophic)
63. **54650-50** (Orchiopexy, Abdominal Approach), **Q53.211** (Nondescent, testicle, bilateral, abdominal)
65. **50520** (Fistula, Closure, Kidney)
67. **53215** (Urethrectomy, Total, Male)
69. **53270** (Skene's Gland, Excision)
71. **55400** (Vasovasorrhaphy)
73. **54600** (Repair, Testis, Torsion)
75. **54056** (Destruction, Lesion, Penis, Cryosurgery)
77. **55100** (Abscess, Scrotum, Incision and Drainage)

Reports

79. Report 36: **52332-50** or **52332-RT** and **52332-LT** (Cystourethroscopy, Insertion, Indwelling Ureteral Stent)
81. Report 38: **53445** (Insertion, Prosthesis, Urethral Sphincter), **R32** (Incontinence), **Z85.46** (History, personal, malignant neoplasm, prostate)
83. Report 82: **52630** (Transurethral Procedure, Prostate, Resection)

85. Report 84: **53852** (Transurethral Procedure, Prostate, Thermotherapy, Radiofrequency), **76872** (Ultrasound, rectal)

CHAPTER 21: REPRODUCTIVE, INTERSEX SURGERY, FEMALE GENITAL SYSTEM, AND MATERNITY CARE AND DELIVERY

Theory

Female Genital Terminology

1. d
3. h
5. b
7. m
9. c
11. j
13. f

Maternity Care and Delivery Terminology

15. e
17. g
19. f
21. j
23. l
25. o
27. i
29. n
31. introitus
33. colpocentesis
35. False
37. colposcope
39. loop electrode excision procedure
41. hysterectomy
43. Radiology
45. Oviduct/Ovary
47. trimesters
49. estimated date (of) delivery
51. E/M

Practical

53. **57400** (Dilation, Vagina)
55. **56441** (Adhesions, Labial, Lysis)
57. **58558** (Hysteroscopy, Surgical with Biopsy)
59. **58920** (Ovary, Wedge Resection)
61. **58800-LT** (Cyst, Ovarian, Incision and Drainage)
63. **59514** (Cesarean Delivery, Delivery Only)
65. **59020** (Fetal Contraction Stress Test)
67. **56440** (Marsupialization, Cyst, Bartholin's Gland)
69. **57065** (Destruction, Lesion, Vagina, Extensive)

Reports

71. Report 28: **59409** (Vaginal Delivery, Delivery Only), **O76** (Delivery, complicated, by, fetal, heart rate or rhythm [abnormal]), **O66.0** (Delivery, complicated, by, obstructed labor, due to, dystocia, shoulder), **O70.1** (Delivery, complicated, by, laceration, perineum, second degree), **Z37.0** (Outcome of delivery, single, liveborn).

    Note: You report the delivery only because by reading this note you have no idea if the delivering physician was her regular obstetrician before and after delivery care.

73. Report 30: **59000** (Amniocentesis, Diagnostic), **O09.293** (Pregnancy, complicated by, poor obstetric history NEC), **Z36.89** (Screening [for], antenatal, of mother), **Z87.448** (History, personal, disease or disorder, urinary system NEC)

CHAPTER 22: ENDOCRINE AND NERVOUS SYSTEMS

Theory

Endocrine System Terminology

1. c
3. f
5. d
7. g
9. h
11. b

Nervous System Terminology

13. g
15. h
17. b
19. d

Practical

21. **60000** (Thyroid Gland, Cyst, Incision and Drainage)
23. **64840** (Suture, Nerve)
25. **64831** (Repair, Nerve, Suture), **69990** (Operating Microscope)
27. **62322** (Injection, Spinal Cord, Anesthetic)
29. **61619** (Skull Base Surgery, Dura, Repair of Cerebrospinal Fluid Leak)
31. **63030** (Hemilaminectomy), **63035** (Hemilaminectomy)

Reports

33. Report 43: **63030-RT** (Hemilaminectomy), **M51.16** (Displacement, intervertebral disc, lumbar region, with neuritis, radiculitis, radiculopathy or sciatica)

CHAPTER 23: EYE, OCULAR ADNEXA, AUDITORY, AND OPERATING MICROSCOPE

Theory

Eye and Ocular Adnexa Terminology

1. a
3. b

5. c
7. d
9. i
11. g
13. k
15. f
17. d
19. h
21. j

Auditory System Terminology

23. g
25. n
27. h
29. i
31. k
33. a
35. c
37. l

Practical

39. **67570-RT** (Decompression, Optic Nerve)
41. **69620-LT** (Myringoplasty)
43. **69661-LT** (Stapedectomy, with Footplate Drill Out)

Reports

45. Report 85: **66720-RT** (Glaucoma, Cryotherapy), **H40.10X3** (Glaucoma, open angle)
47. Report 87: **66984-RT** (Cataract, Removal/Extraction, Extracapsular)

CHAPTER 24: RADIOLOGY

Theory

1. c
3. b
5. a
7. b
9. f
11. a
13. e
15. i
17. h
19. j
21. c

Practical

23. **78499** (Unlisted Services and Procedures, Nuclear Medicine, Heart)
25. -26

27. **75705** (Angiography, Spinal Artery)
29. **70130** (X-Ray, Mastoids)
31. **70542** (Magnetic Resonance Imaging [MRI], Diagnostic, Neck)
33. **73502** (X-Ray, Hip)
35. **76098** (X-Ray, Specimen/Surgical)
37. **99222** for initial observation care (Evaluation and Management, Hospital); **70450** for CT Scan without mention of contrast (CT Scan, without Contrast), **76516** for A-scan (Ultrasound, Eye, Biometry); **77261** for therapeutic radiation (Radiation Therapy, Planning); **77402** simple radiation delivery (Radiation Therapy, Treatment Delivery, Single); **77427** for weekly radiology therapy management (Radiation Therapy, Treatment Management, Weekly)
39. **76604** (Ultrasound, Chest); **71550** for the MRI (Magnetic Resonance Imaging [MRI], Diagnostic, Chest); **33020** for the pericardiotomy (Pericardiotomy, Removal, Clot)
41. **73092** (X-Ray, Arm, Upper)
43. **77002** (Fluoroscopy, Needle Biopsy)
45. **76872** (Ultrasound, Rectal)
47. **72240** (Myelography, Spine, Cervical)
49. **70140** (X-Ray, Facial Bones)
51. **74019** (X-Ray, Abdomen)
53. **75870** (Venography, Sagittal Sinus), **G08** (Thrombosis, sinus, intracranial)
55. **37252** (Ultrasound, Non-Coronary, Intravascular), **I70.1** (Stenosis, artery, renal)

Reports

57. Report 45: **71045-26** (X-Ray, Chest), **R07.9** (Pain, chest [central])
59. Report 47: **70480-26** (CT Scan, without Contrast, Orbit), **H57.12** (Pain, eye)
61. Report 49: **74018-26** (X-Ray, Abdomen), **E46** (Malnutrition)
63. Report 51: **74160-26** (CT, with Contrast, Abdomen), **R94.5** (Findings, abnormal, inconclusive, function study, liver)
65. Report 53: **78451-26** (Myocardial, Perfusion Imaging), **R07.9** (Pain[s], chest [central]), **R06.02** (Short, breath)

CHAPTER 25: PATHOLOGY/LABORATORY

Theory

1. Surgery
3. presence, amount or amount, presence
5. section
7. one

Practical

9. **84520** (Urea Nitrogen, Quantitative), **84295** (Sodium), **84132** (Potassium), **82565** (Creatinine, Blood), **84550** (Uric Acid, Blood), **E86.0** (Dehydration), **M25.50** (Pain, joint), **R50.9** (Fever)

Note: The Blood Urea Nitrogen (BUN) is part of the blood chemistry for this patient, and there are two codes for blood as the source of the sample—**84520** and **84525**. Although there are other CPT codes to identify urea nitrogen, the source of the sample for those codes is the urine (**84540, 84545**).

11. **80076** (Blood Tests, Panels, Hepatic Function), **80061** (Blood Tests, Panels, Lipid Panel), **E78.5** (Hyperlipidemia)
13. **80162** (Therapeutic Drug Assay, Digoxin), **I48.20** (Fibrillation, atrial or auricular, chronic)

Reports

15. Report 55: **88305** Urinary Bladder (Pathology, Surgical, Gross and Micro Exam, Level IV), **D09.0** (Table of Neoplasms: Neoplasm, bladder, Ca in-situ)
17. Report 57: **88304** Intervertebral Disc (Pathology, Surgical, Gross and Micro Exam, Level III), **M51.26** (Displacement, intervertebral disc, lumbar region)
19. Report 59: **88305** Muscle (Pathology, Surgical, Gross and Micro Exam, Level IV), **M79.18** (Myalgia, site specified NEC)
21. Report 61: **88304** Skin Cyst (Pathology, Surgical, Gross and Micro Exam, Level III), **L72.9** (Cyst, skin)
23. Report 63: **88307** Liver (Pathology, Surgical, Gross and Micro Exam, Level V), **E66.01** (Obesity, morbid), **K76.0** (Fatty, liver NEC)
25. Report 65: **88309** Lung Lobe (Pathology, Surgical, Gross and Micro Exam, Level VI), **J85.2** (Abscess, lung)
27. Report 67: **88104** (Cytopathology, Fluids, Washings, Brushings, Smears), **J90** (Effusion, pleura)

CHAPTER 26: MEDICINE

Theory

1. m
3. h
5. n
7. i
9. g
11. l
13. a
15. g
17. f
19. a
21. c
23. hearing test
25. stimulation of the cochlea to measure electrical activity
27. studying the capillaries of the eyes
29. a device for detecting color blindness
31. cornea and sclera together forming one organ
33. the thick outer coat of the eye, mostly white and opaque

Practical

35. **95052 x 2** (Allergy Tests, Patch, Photo Patch)
37. **92341** (Spectacle Services, Fitting, Spectacles)
39. **92534** (Nystagmus Tests, Optokinetic)
41. **91034** (Esophagus, Acid Reflux Tests)
43. **90880** (Hypnotherapy)
45. **92626** (Evaluation, Auditory Function, Function of Auditory Implant)
47. **90940** (Hemodialysis, Blood Flow Study)
49. **93503** (Cardiac Catheterization, Insertion, Flow Directed Catheter, Swan Ganz)
51. **94003** (Ventilation Assist), **J96.00** (Failure, respiration, respiratory, acute)
53. **99152, 99153** (Sedation, Moderate)
55. **90471** (Administration, Immunization, One Vaccine/Toxoid), **90472** (Administration, Immunization, each additional Vaccine/Toxoid)
57. **I21.19** (Infarct, myocardium, ST elevation, inferior [inferolateral]), **I23.1** (Defect, atrial septal, following acute myocardial infarction)

Reports

59. Report 68: **99203** (Office and/or Other Outpatient Services, New Patient), **I25.10** (Arteriosclerosis, coronary [artery]), **I10** (Hypertension), **N63.20** (Mass, breast), **Z95.1** (Status [post], aortocoronary bypass), **Z79.890** (Long-term, hormone replacement [postmenopausal]), **Z82.49** (History, family, disease or disorder [of], cardiovascular NEC), **Z80.3** (History, family, malignant neoplasm [of], breast)
61. Report 70: **99242** (Consultation, Office and/or Other Outpatient)
63. Report 72: **none,** as the admission is part of the surgical package
65. Report 74: **19307-LT** (Mastectomy, Modified Radical), **C50.912** (Table of Neoplasms: Neoplasm, breast, Primary)
67. Report 76: **99252-57** (Consultation, Inpatient) modifier -57 indicates the decision for major surgery, **I97.89** (Complication, circulatory system, post-procedural), **M79.606** (Pain, limb, lower)
69. Report 78: **32554** (Thoracentesis), **J90** (Effusion, pleural)

    Note: The report indicated the patient was developing respiratory failure; if the failure was confirmed, the diagnosis would be reported with **J96.00** (Failure, respiration, respiratory, acute).
71. Report 80: **94060** (Spirometry), **94729** (Pulmonology, Diagnostic, Carbon Monoxide Diffusion Capacity), **99070** (Supplies, Materials) for the bronchodilator

CHAPTER 27: INPATIENT CODING

Theory

1. Inpatient
3. Outpatient
5. False
7. False
9. a

11. b
13. c
15. c

Sequencing Exercises

Cases of Principal Diagnosis and Other Diagnoses

17. Principal diagnosis: congestive heart failure
    Other diagnoses: none
19. Principal diagnosis: postoperative hemorrhage
    Other diagnoses: ovarian cancer, primary
21. Principal diagnosis: third-degree burn to arm/stomach (either the arm or stomach could be sequenced first)
    Other diagnoses: second-degree burn thigh
23. Principal diagnosis: dehydration
    Other diagnoses: gastroenteritis
    Pregnancy is reported with a V code for incidental state.

Principal Diagnosis

25. Principal diagnosis and code: Right posterior and anterior communicating artery aneurysm **I67.1** (Aneurysm, brain)
    Other diagnosis and code:
    Right otitis externa **H60.91** (Otitis, externa)
    Procedure: **03VG0ZZ** Right craniotomy for clipping of arterial aneurysm (Restriction, Artery, Intracranial)

